THE HALL OF MIRRORS

How to Change Life Patterns and Avoid Toxic Relationships

By Kath Twigg

First published 2018
Published by Forward Thinking Publishing
Text © Kath Twigg 2018

A catalogue record for this book is available from
the British Library.

ISBN: 978-0-9934652-7-7

For my amazing Dad,
whose love moved Heaven and Earth,
and for my wonderful husband,
who helped me to break the pattern.

Contents

Introduction

Chapters:

Contents

INTRODUCTION

"Every generation
Blames the one before
And all of their frustrations
Come beating on your door

I know that I'm a prisoner
To all my father held so dear
I know that I'm a hostage
To all his hopes and fears
I just wish I could have told him
In the living years"

Mike and the Mechanics 'The Living Years'

I have titled this book 'The Hall of Mirrors' because relationships always remind me of the fairground experience of seeing yourself from all angles in a room full of mirrors, as though echoing into the past. The reflection comes from a single source but repeats, over and over. Miraculously, if you remove yourself from the room, the pattern disappears.

The quote from Mike and the Mechanics at the head of this chapter has always seemed particularly poignant to me-we can see the seeds of our experiences in past relationships but rarely do we get the chance to put these things right. Whether the genesis of your pattern lies in a relationship with someone who is still living or who has passed away, understanding what happened and why is the key to your journey towards a healthier life.

1

What follows is an account of my experiences with toxic relationships and my efforts to overcome them. It's a journey through which I learned to love and respect myself and to find a peaceful and fulfilling existence, but only after years of unhappiness. It was first written as a piece of therapeutic writing, a process which helped me to make sense of my experiences and to move on. Latterly it has evolved into much more; given my training and experience I am naturally interested in human behaviour and the potential for change and improvement. I am also concerned that the inter-relationship between life patterns and toxic relationships is not widely understood; I'd like to provide an explanation and challenge some misconceptions.

In essence, the subject of this book is my struggle with 'traumatic bonding', sometimes called the 'Stockholm Syndrome'. It is the reason why people become trapped in unhealthy relationships and the answer to the question - why do they stay? - which is often asked of victims of domestic abuse.

There are many misconceptions about the issues which are the subject of this book. There is a school of popular psychology in which the phrase 'love addict' is typically applied to people like myself who become trapped in toxic relationships; it is a concept I wish to challenge and redefine through the telling of my story and the techniques I have developed. 'Love addiction' (a phrase I will not use again) is said to apply more widely to women than to men and my concern is that, as currently described, it may reinforce the stereotype of women as over-emotional and unstable. It is also at risk of trivialising what is a complex and destructive phenomenon. This runs the risk of pathologising victims and survivors of abuse and blaming them for their experiences. In turn, survivors can blame themselves; I have heard people describe themselves as 'attracting the wrong partners', a concept which concerns me greatly. Such thinking resonates with the tendency of abusers to blame victims and fosters wider misunderstanding.

Toxic relationships have nothing to do with love. Essentially a very personal and somewhat indefinable emotion, love is an inherently positive and affirming connection between human beings which embodies, for example, compassion, kindness and selflessness. Compare this to the destructive, dangerous and negative experiences which accompany abusive relationships and it is difficult to see how these bear any resemblance to love.

I have therefore developed my original work to incorporate more explanation of what can happen and why and added some exercises based on my experiences and knowledge which you can use to help you to escape and to avoid similar experiences

I have also devised a group programme which I can deliver for you as a course or retreat. My contact details are included at the end of this book.

I want to be clear that people who find themselves subject to abuse (either male or female) are *not* responsible for the behaviour of their abusers, nor are they flawed in some way which causes them to "attract" the wrong people. As my story illustrates, it is the pattern of staying in unhealthy relationships and trying to put things right, rather than accepting that nothing will change and walking away which needs to be tackled. This pattern comes from early experience or trauma and consequent feelings of low self-worth and insecurity, resulting in vain attempts to fulfil deep personal need.

Traumatic bonding forms and reinforces habitual behaviour, undermining self-confidence and leading to unwise choices and unhappiness, which can repeat throughout your life. As such it is amenable to change given the right techniques and approaches. My message is ultimately that changing yourself and your behavioural patterns is the only enduring way to overcome such challenges. We are all adults, free to make rational choices with the right support.

There is a range of support systems and interventions for victims and survivors of abuse. However, I am well aware that there is a group of people who, for whatever reason, feel unable to access them. This leaves them doubly isolated and vulnerable. If this is you, then I am particularly interested in helping you to find some inspiration and encouragement through my story.

We all need healthy relationships, whether with life partners, wider family or friends; they are a pre-requisite for a happy life. To suggest that we need to recognise our self-worth before we can achieve such relationships is not to imply that only 'well balanced' people can form successful partnerships, or that a period of enforced loneliness is necessary before we can achieve a peaceful and fulfilling life.   What is important is that people who have experienced instability, unhappiness and abuse should gain support and guidance before entering into life partnerships which may be based on unhealthy foundations.

The first step in this process is to recognise where things have gone wrong in the past and why this has happened.   In the course of my reflections and the process of writing this book, I came to recognise that for much of my life since early adolescence I had been preoccupied with an ideal of romantic love which seemed always to elude me. I became distracted from work, my family, friends and other obligations by its pursuit, devastated when inevitably my hopes were dashed, and overwhelmed with the desire to put things right when the situation was hopeless; all recognised aspects of traumatic bonding.

As a consequence, I endured years of misery and depression which inevitably affected the lives of those closest to me. It's important to acknowledge that, although my story has a happy ending, the pursuit of romantic love is not, in itself, the point.   Once we decide to tackle the roots of unhealthy relationships and recognise that we all have the right to be happy and loved, healthy relationships naturally follow.

Ultimately, I believe that the most effective action any survivor of toxic relationships can take is to recognise that they cannot change others' behaviour but they *can* change their own and make themselves safer with the help of the right people and resources. I have tried to tell my story with as much honesty and self-reflection as possible as an illustration both of the extreme difficulty people such as myself can face in trying to break away, and as a message of hope that it can be done. I have included the spiritual components as an honest account of my experience; though some readers may find them difficult to accept, they are a vital element in my personal development and to leave them out would present an incomplete picture.

4

My perspective is inevitably that of a heterosexual woman, though toxic and dysfunctional relationships can exist between same or opposite sex life partners, colleagues, line managers and employees and wider family members. They can be found across and between cultures and within minority groups. Many victims of abuse encounter several types of dysfunctional relationships, as in my case. My experience has taught me that the pattern is similar no matter what the nature of the relationship and its resolution lies in the recognition that we always have a choice to break free, recognise our self-worth and make clearer and more insightful decisions about our lives.

This is a complex subject and tackling it requires strength and dedication-walking away from your most recent unhealthy relationship is only the first step. Here you will find no quick fix techniques or panacea for life challenges. My struggle against the effects of my life pattern has been so hard and quite literally almost fatal. I made many mistakes, suffered unnecessarily and finally had to look inside to find the answer. My story illustrates just how complicated and multi-faceted life patterns and their effects can become. What is important is to recognise the genesis of our behaviour, to identify *why* we behave as we do in entering into and remaining in situations where others abuse, stifle or exert power over us. Once we know that, for example, we are trying repeatedly to fix a childhood trauma, we can begin to see our lives more clearly and look for alternatives.

Even if you have not directly experienced abuse, I believe that anyone who has experienced unhappy, unstable or unfulfilling relationships can benefit from my story, especially if you also choose to complete the suggested exercises which accompany it.

Ultimately, if we behave out of neediness or fear we are less likely to make wise and informed decisions. I hope that in reading my story you will come to realise why acting out of love for yourself is vitally important to recovery from the torture of destructive behavioural patterns and the key to a happier, more balanced life. Here is my story, in the hope that it will help others to find a way out of the pain.

If you have experienced or are still involved in toxic relationships, I encourage you to complete the simple exercises included at the end of the book. They will help you to see more clearly what you want and deserve from life and enable you to act more compassionately towards yourself.

1.

PATTERNS

"I'm the voice you never listen to and I had
to break your heart to make you see,
He's the one who will be missing you,
and you'll only miss the man that
you wanted him to be,
Turn the radio on"

Chely Wright, 'shut up and drive'

For twelve years of my precious and only life I had a relationship with a man who systematically removed everything that made it worth living. He insulted and criticised me, refused to go out with me, rubbished my career, my beliefs and preferences and rejected my family and friends. He displayed bizarre and irrational behaviour and there were instances of physical abuse. Repeatedly I tried everything I could to persuade and encourage him to show the slightest hint of affection, reassurance or interest; to become, once again, the man I thought I had met, the man I wanted him to be.

Somehow I seemed addicted to this struggle, unable to let go and desperate to prolong the agony in the name of irrational hope and expectation. I felt that, if I could only find the right words or do the right things, he would change into the true love of my life and I would finally be happy.

Why did I stay when anyone with a shred of self-respect would have walked away?

I stayed because I became locked into a pattern of attempting to change my partner rather than recognising that I needed to leave. This pattern typically happens as a result of traumatic and damaging early experiences. For example, children of alcohol dependent parents will repeatedly try to 'put things right'. Trapped in a difficult and chaotic situation, they make frequent and invariably futile attempts to change their parents' behaviour, believing that if they can succeed they will find happiness.

In later life, such experiences can cause adults to repeat the pattern of trying to change others to find happiness. Where more secure individuals would immediately recognise the signs and signals of a dysfunctional relationship, adults who are insecure become over-attached, lose objectivity and fear loss. In consequence they fall into the familiar pattern of trying too hard to please, attempting to reason despite evidence that nothing can change and rationalising the situation with false hope.

I had a somewhat strange and confusing childhood. My parents were not alcohol dependent; they were tee-total, committed Methodists and well regarded by their peers. Ostensibly I had a respectable, mainstream childhood in a lower middle-class family. I was never physically abused, my material needs were always catered for and I was regarded as an intelligent child with good prospects. Yet beneath the surface, my life was far from happy.

As a young child I was isolated from my mother, whose constant ill health was, I suspect, partly a product of the over-protection of her mother, who never recovered from the trauma of losing her son, my mother's only sibling, in the Second World War. My early childhood was therefore characterised by the ever-present fear that my mother was going to die, projected from my maternal grandmother who lived with us, combined with a prevailing sense that I was 'in the way', or at least a constant source of annoyance. I was berated for making a noise which might give my mother a headache, leaving doors open as she might be in a draught and trying to sit on her knee as she had 'bad legs'. Attempts to bring friends into the house or garden were met with embarrassing rebuttals from my grandmother.

At a vulnerable time in my life, therefore, instead of developing a balanced and happy personality, I felt confused, rejected and had little sense of who I was.

I have two much older brothers who went their own very different ways. We were never a coherent family, the age difference between siblings meaning that I was the embarrassing younger sister when they were adolescents, and we were not close. Strangely, my older brothers were treated with much more respect than me, almost like honoured guests. Activities which were viewed as an annoyance from me were seen differently when my brothers were involved. I remember one confusing incident when my middle brother was playing music in a room adjacent to the kitchen, where I was also present. My grandmother shouted for me to turn the music down as it would give my mother a headache. I pointed out that the music was being played by my brother, not me, at which point my grandmother became highly embarrassed and started apologising profusely to my brother. It seemed that even music became annoying if played by me.

Only in adulthood, as I have grown closer to my brothers, have I understood from them that they also found our family environment confusing and odd. My middle brother would never bring girlfriends to the house as he was too embarrassed. He played in a pop group and was frequently derided by my father for being late home. My older brother recounted incidents where friends were made to feel unwelcome and his early girlfriends were disliked and rejected. We all have confusing and embarrassing memories of my mother's attention-seeking behaviour over illness, her frequent fainting when she found situations difficult to handle and her preoccupation with herself.

Although I don't remember feeling particularly unwanted as a child, there were hints that I was an 'afterthought' and unexpected.

Even in early childhood, then, I was isolated and unhappy. My childlike enthusiasm was repressed, my friends were disapproved of and discouraged and I lived in an atmosphere of fear projected from adults in the household. Although, on one level, I believe I knew I was loved, I didn't *feel* loved. My resultant behaviour was attention seeking and self-conscious. I never really knew how to behave and found myself trying to copy others, obscuring my natural personality and suffering from anxiety and the need for approval, which manifested in hyper-activity and awkwardness.

Eventually, my grandmother developed Alzheimer's disease. For several years, as her condition deteriorated, I remember night after night of lost sleep as she would wander and become anxious. Often, I would hide under the covers, petrified that she would come into my room, listening to my parents and grandfather trying to placate her. Strangely through my grandmother's illness my mother looked after her with great care, her own illnesses forgotten.

If I had any love for my grandmother, it evaporated quickly during this period. Her eventual death was a great relief and I shed no tears.

The saving grace was my father, a kind and intelligent man who loved children and who, despite the long hours he worked, devoted himself to me. He read to me at bedtime, talked endlessly to me about his beliefs and philanthropy and provided me with fun and laughter. As a result, I was given a lifeline, a foil to the repression, guilt and negativity from elsewhere. His demonstrations of love and appreciation allowed me to flourish academically and, despite the context of my awkward personality, I developed a strong moral conscience, a set of beliefs and an ability to articulate them which provided me with much needed strength, though there was a down-side. In a way I became my father; lacking the confidence to make clear decisions about my preferences and desires I would often make choices based on his. Thus, I learned to look for approval and validation in the outside world, rather than within myself, making life choices in the hope of pleasing others, rather than decisions based on what I really wanted to achieve.

In my early teens, disaster struck. Developing into a young woman, I began seeking independence, exploring sexuality and developing relationships with the opposite sex. Immediately my relationship with my father changed. I was no longer the obedient and adoring little girl with whom he felt safe. He became controlling and aggressive, critical of my lifestyle and behaviour. The shock of losing his affection and approval in this way set a pattern for my life. I would repeatedly be convinced that I had found happiness and security, only to see it dissipate in the cruellest way.

I remember many years of trying to engage my father in conversation, attempting to explain that I was simply growing up and seeking more freedom. I recall a moment when I could hold in my anger towards my father no longer; I began to scream "why, just tell me why?" He would not listen and he would not answer. The overwhelming memory of this protracted period of my adolescence is of my inability to reason with my father. Alone in my room, I cried endlessly. My school work deteriorated, further enraging my father. I needed love and support, a listening ear and a sense of encouragement; things could have been so different.

In desperation I wrote my father a letter explaining how I felt and what I needed. In anger he threw it on the fire unopened with the words "you can write and write, but it will make no difference." I was devastated. In that moment I felt I had lost him.

I have said that people who are insecure and have low self-esteem fear loss and rejection above all things. Their very existence as personalities becomes dependent on the approval of others; they believe themselves nothing without this. I became more and more dependent on relationships with young men, seeking the elusive feeling of being loved, mistakenly confused with sexual attraction. At the age of seventeen I became pregnant. The father of my child was a handsome man I met on holiday. From a very different background to mine, initially I found him exciting and charismatic. I accepted his excessive use of alcohol and innate aggression without question, facets of his unfettered lifestyle. My father hated him. When I became pregnant my father was incandescent with anger. Six months after my seventeenth birthday I became a married woman.

Over the next few years my life changed dramatically. My son was born one month before my eighteenth birthday. I adored him from the moment I saw him, I felt a sense of overwhelming love and protection, and an ever-present fear for his safety. My relationship with my husband Joe was turbulent and unhappy from the start. My handsome and charismatic partner became aggressive and selfish and for the second time in my life I lost the feeling of love from a man on whom I had come to depend for my emotional wellbeing. Half of our income was spent on alcohol and I learned much later that throughout our marriage of eighteen years he was constantly unfaithful, repeatedly emphasising that he didn't like being married. I was young and immature, not ready to be married with a child, and desperately unhappy.

Despite my unhappiness and the clear recognition that I should leave, I found myself unable to let go. I tried to reason, cried many tears and worked hard to keep up a respectable facade. I realise now that I was hoping desperately that my husband would 'see the light', realise how much he loved me and change into a different person. Instead, he seemed to live his life despite me and our son. At times he would behave abominably in the company of friends and acquaintances, leaving me racked with embarrassment. Our often violent arguments frequently resulted in threats from one or both of us to end the relationship, yet afterwards I invariably found myself pleading with him to stay, terrified of being alone.

Our relationship sometimes degenerated into physical violence, and neither of us was faithful. At times I would become hysterical with frustration; the irony, once again, of asking "why?" and not being heard, was not lost on me, but still I stayed. I began to fantasise about separation and divorce yet couldn't muster the courage to leave.

Following the death of my grandmother, the birth of my son and the traumas with my father, my relationship with my mother had begun to improve. She and I became closer and my parents lived near-by and helped with my son, thank goodness as his life at home was traumatic enough. My father remained distant from me, yet he loved my son dearly and lavished on him the attention I remembered from early childhood, and my mother cared for my son when I eventually went to work.

My self-esteem was very low. I saw virtually everyone I encountered as more 'worthy' or 'respectable' than me. I was self-conscious and full of guilt, shame and a sense of failure. I decided to go back to studying, having worked for a couple of years as a low ranking civil servant. I looked into the funding situation for university and discovered that, even though I was married, due to my age I was required to submit information about my father's income in order to obtain a grant. His reaction to my request for help was the final straw in my earthly relationship with my father. He resented the intrusion into his private affairs, questioned my decision to go to university as a 'married woman' (even though this had been his greatest wish for me when I was a child) and made the process very difficult. His reaction spoke volumes; I was another man's wife, a disappointment; I felt he had written me off and we were distanced even further.

Shortly afterwards my father became ill, developing pre-senile dementia. I felt so deeply for my mother, she had nursed her own mother with dementia and now she had to cope with the loss of her husband, still only in his late fifties, to that terrible disease. Mercifully my father passed away shortly afterwards; I felt I had lost him for the last time.

Over the following years I studied hard and gained a good degree. I began to work in the social work field and soon found myself taking a higher degree and seeking promotion, constantly trying to prove myself. My relationship with my husband was still traumatic, yet I felt trapped and helpless to leave. I hid the traumas from my friends and colleagues, pretended all was well, whilst secretly feeling inferior and shameful; everyone around me seemed to have happy relationships and respectable lives. Despite my hard work, nothing I had achieved made me happy.

My marriage ended suddenly. I discovered that my husband had been having a six-year affair. I was furious but hardly in a position to judge as I had not been faithful myself. My feelings were like a roller coaster; anger, relief, fear, grief and confusion. There was even a sense that I didn't want the marriage to end, yet I somehow found the strength to see it through. Finally, it was over.

Ultimately, I felt a profound sense of gratitude, believed that my life would improve beyond recognition and waited for Mr Right to come along. I should have taken a deep breath, stabilised my life and that of my son, got to know myself and enjoyed the freedom. I did none of these things; my son was due to go to university in a few months and I was petrified of living alone. I told myself I had to meet someone before he left.

I had a friend, a dear friend; his name was Steve. We worked together, had lots in common and he made me laugh. We had been intimate, but unlike any relationship I had ever had with a man, I never saw him as a potential partner, and I knew that my son wasn't keen on him. We were both in relationships with other people. When my marriage ended we agreed to meet each other, but nothing more.

Two months after I separated from my first husband I met Sam.

2.

SAM

*"All of us have blocks of habit energy inside us.
Habit energy is the unconscious energy that causes
us to repeat the same behaviour thousands of times.
Habit energy pushes us to run, to always be doing
something, to be lost in thoughts of the past or the
future, and to blame others for our suffering.
It interferes with our ability to be happy
in the present moment."*

Thich Nhat Hanh, 'Silence'

Sam and I were introduced by mutual friends. Twelve years older than me, tall and looking older than his years, Sam appeared charming and cultured. Recently separated from his wife of many years, there was nothing clandestine or guilt-ridden about our liaison. My son met him and approved.

At first I was unsure of Sam. On our first date he behaved impeccably, taking me to a local restaurant. I had been so full of anticipation yet found myself un-attracted to him. I couldn't help noticing that, despite his polished social skills, Sam rarely looked me in the eye during conversation. The morning after our first meeting, I awoke in floods of tears; something was just not right.

Later that day, a large bunch of red roses arrived from Sam. I

15

began to feel better; no one had ever treated me so kindly. I rang him to say "thanks" and he was gracious and flattering. My earlier reservations and intuitive feelings side-lined, I agreed to meet him again.

Our relationship took off and I became captivated with a sense of romance. It was clear that we were very different. Sam's views were morally and politically dissimilar to mine, he seemed somewhat old fashioned and tended to spurn my liberal politics and outlook. From very early on there were comments about his dislike of my job and he had a tendency to jealousy; these things I dismissed, quite literally seduced by his declarations of love and outward charm. My family met and liked him.

Within six months we took a holiday to Greece, during which Sam asked me to marry him. I knew it was too soon, certainly for me and probably for both of us, yet I accepted. During the year that followed I moved into his house and put mine on sale. There were frequent moments of conflict which should have caused me to end the relationship. Following a night out with old friends he stood on the landing screaming "where the hell have you been?" There was more derision about my job, criticism of my clothes, dislike of my friends. Yet I convinced myself somehow that he was the love of my life, and I persevered. I thought his background and demeanour would make me respectable, that finally I had a relationship to equal that of my friends and colleagues. It was as if I could not trust myself to command the respect of others in my own right. How could I have been so shallow and so wrong?

We went through a traumatic period of disagreements leading up to our wedding, which I attributed to the stress of the event, never considering that we might not be compatible. Just less than two years after my first marriage ended, I married Sam. Our honeymoon, in the Caribbean, began well. The inevitable deterioration came, when one of the staff paid me a compliment, and Sam became enraged. He accused me of dressing provocatively and insisted on making a complaint to the management of the hotel about the employee. I was overcome with anger and embarrassment. His jealousy was irrational, his attack on me completely unjustified.

Although we went through the motions, the honeymoon was ruined.

Shortly after we returned, Sam lost his job and was quickly offered another in the south of England. This required a move and a change of job for me and moved me away from my family and the area I had lived in all my life.

If there had been vestiges of the charming Sam in our relationship before our move, they completely disappeared once we started our new life. He became arrogant, controlling and obstructive. I found myself incredulous, constantly demanding an explanation for his complete change in character. Once again, I heard myself demanding "why?" and receiving no rational explanation. Once again, I was losing the love of a man on whom I had depended for my emotional security; once again I was losing my father. I became profoundly depressed. All that sustained me was my new job, which I loved and which gave me an essential sense of self-worth. For the first time in my life I resorted to anti-depressants.

Signs of violence from Sam began to surface; once a slap across the face, once a lunge which I managed to dodge. The criticism of my clothes continued; I tried to find more conservative items to please him but nothing was good enough. He described me as looking like "an overgrown schoolgirl" so I cut my very long hair short. Sam repeatedly planned visits to his family and friends, whilst avoiding mine. My family and friends were clearly not welcome in our home. Whilst outwardly maintaining a charming façade, Sam would privately preface their visits with negative comments and make clear his disapproval. I found myself dreading their arrival and constantly on edge during visits, fearing that Sam would cause embarrassment. Their telephone calls to me were interrupted by demands and embarrassing comments from Sam, which I tried to dismiss or cover with light-hearted comments. Home was not a safe or comfortable place, I cried repeatedly.

Sam refused to go out in the evenings and our social life became almost non-existent. I found myself doing all the shopping, cooking and household chores.

Distanced geographically from my family and friends, I found myself also cast adrift emotionally. My regular phone calls home diminished in frequency as Sam's disapproval and rude interruptions made them unbearable. Finally defeated by frustration and embarrassment, I refused to answer the phone, insisting that if Sam answered he was to say I was out. Ultimately it didn't matter, in the end no one rang for me.

Over the next few years, Sam's behaviour deteriorated further. He became self-obsessed and convinced that he was suffering serious illnesses. He constantly berated me for not being understanding. Some days he refused to get out of bed. Eventually he decided to leave work and take up his modest pension. He suggested a move to the south coast and despite his dislike of my job, encouraged me to take up a promotion. Having always loved the sea, and thinking that the change would improve our relationship, I agreed. The move took me away from the job I enjoyed, removed me further from the people I loved and isolated me even more.

We lived in a beautiful place high on a hill with the kind of views I always dreamt about. I would open the curtains in the morning and see boats on the river. The view was never the same, with each change in the weather the light revealed a new masterpiece. The sky was so clear the stars took your breath away. I had always wanted to live by the sea, now I lived within a short distance of some of the most spectacular coastline in Britain. And I had never been so unhappy.

After our move, it became clear that Sam was not going to change. He stopped contributing to day to day expenses, which I covered from my salary, did nothing to help in the house despite his retirement, and joined a local golf club, where he spent much of his time. He refused to help me decorate our new house and would not agree to employ someone to help with the refurbishment. I did what I could myself. Despite the beauty of our surroundings we never spent time exploring the area together; there was always a reason why Sam didn't want to go. I knew, of course that this was simply part of his campaign to deny me activities which he knew would give me pleasure, yet I stayed.

My new job was demanding and my new boss turned out to be an extreme bully. For several years I was under severe pressure at work, which almost ended my career. I had been warned by colleagues that my new boss had a reputation for bullying and had left a trail of destruction in his wake. I was aware that, after his arrival in my new area, several members of the senior management team, which I was about to join, had taken long term sickness absence or been suspended. I discovered that the devastation did not stop there. Many middle managers and other staff were similarly affected and there was a palpable atmosphere of fear.

I quickly discovered that my new boss's approach was calculated to provide him with maximum power. He kept every scrap of evidence of interactions with colleagues, required signatures indicating that all policy documents and regulations had been read, and applied extreme pressure for his objectives to be fulfilled to the letter, with the purpose of enhancing his reputation. He cultivated unprofessional relationships with the unions and some members of the Board. His actions were calculated to allow him to discipline or side-line any colleague who stepped out of line by holding them to account in minute detail, encouraging grievance procedures against staff he saw as a threat and using the agency's regulations against them. Staff taking out grievances and attempting to challenge him were subjected to the most extreme pressure.

The result was an unstable and chaotic organisation where litigious process, internal and external, was rife. No one could be trusted as everyone was in fear.

Having moved from a job which gave me the only sense of self-worth I had experienced for years, I quickly found myself deeply troubled and at odds with my boss. I was horrified at the oppressive management approach I was expected to take and found myself unable to function effectively. Even the most basic task left me anxious and floundering.

As a result, I was unable to perform to the level my boss required. It was clear he wanted me out. Fortunately, I had personal connections with people in positions of influence who held me in high regard. I was able to blow the whistle on what was happening, but not before it had brought me to my knees emotionally and I was forced to take sickness absence for several months.

Sam offered no support, refusing to discuss my work problems. When work colleagues rang me at home, Sam interrupted the phone calls by shouting abuse or insisting he was waiting for a phone call and I was blocking the phone. He seemed to feed off the power he exerted over me in this way; my protestations were to no avail.

Sam's harsh criticism of me continued, and I saw less and less of my family and friends. All intimacy between us had ceased and it was clear that Sam could see no good in me. Whilst I was away from work, Sam became even more controlling. He tried to restrict my movements, complaining when I went out or stayed out for too long, and blocking my car so that I couldn't leave the house. I felt powerless and imprisoned. My life seemed worthless.

I was too ashamed to confide in friends or family, not wishing to be seen as a failure or a burden. I tried to pretend that all was well, a process made easier by my isolation.

I talked to my GP who advised me to leave Sam. I didn't take the advice. Once again, I resorted to anti-depressants. I became so low I considered suicide, yet my efforts to change Sam continued. Against overwhelming evidence that my life was not working, instead of changing my job and leaving my partner, I persevered with both extremely unhealthy situations as though I had no choice, carrying on as though some fixed universal law decreed that it should be so.

This was the lowest point of my life; my isolation was complete, my confidence undermined and the only light relief I could find was from solitary outings to the beach or prolonged shopping trips. I felt that no one could help me and firmly believe that, if events had not dictated otherwise, I would have remained in that situation for the rest of my life.

3.

MESSAGE FROM AN OLD FRIEND

"Reaching no absolute in which to rest
One is always nearer by not keeping still."

Thom Gunn, 'On the Move'

My boss eventually moved on; he was subsequently to lose his new job in a very public way for behaviour similar to that which I had experienced. The episode had left me deeply scarred, and whilst I received an apology and was offered some external support, the approach from my new boss was "we know how awful this was and we're sorry, but let's just get on with the job". I dealt with all of this in my characteristic manner, by driving myself forwards.

I began to enjoy my job again, pushing myself doubly hard to prove my competence, though never stopping to allow myself to recover or to consider what I really wanted.

Despite this improvement, I was weighed down by the burden of my relationship with Sam. There were times when I would drag myself to work, utterly shattered by depression and hopelessness, fighting tears and struggling to centre myself. I somehow managed to keep my secret hidden from the outside world, separating myself into two unequal parts, one a powerless and desperate prisoner of my dysfunctional relationship, the other a capable and confident professional. Eventually, though, it became more and more difficult to cover my tracks and my colleagues began to notice that something was wrong.

We lived in a small, remote village some twenty miles from my office and further still from headquarters, which I was required to visit often for various meetings and events. One morning I was travelling to headquarters for the monthly meeting attended by my peers and chaired by my boss, Jim. As usual I had lost track of time; prone to waking at first light I could have simply got myself together, left the house in plenty of time and arrived at the office without the added pressure of lateness, embarrassment and excuses. Instead I engaged in what had become a pointless yet addictive ritual. Believing that, through sheer persistence, I might finally find the right words to get my message through to Sam, I had once again made a cup of tea, taken it back to bed and begun the process of trying to persuade him to change. The compulsion to proceed with this humiliating and demoralising struggle frequently distorted my sense of priorities, causing me to put off my departure for work until way past the last moment. I could cover my tracks on days when I worked in my own office, making up for morning lateness by working well into the evening, but scheduled meetings were more formal and public, subject to far less flexibility.

As usual, I had failed to take into account the inevitable traffic chaos which surrounds large cities in the morning rush hour. In the fog of desperation which clouded my thoughts in all matters related to Sam, I side-lined any consideration which might distract me from my hopeless mission to gain his attention. Now, sitting in a stagnant traffic queue, I began to panic, knowing that I faced another humiliating experience, picturing with dread my colleagues once again engaged in the business agenda, turning to acknowledge my late entrance.

Finally, the tortuous journey was almost over. As usual, by the time I arrived, most parking spaces were full, and it took a further five minutes to find a place to park then walk through the expansive grounds to the building itself.

By now breathless and harassed, I flew up the stairs and burst into the meeting mumbling something about awful traffic. Although outwardly polite and forgiving, I knew that Jim would later be disapproving and braced myself for the inevitable "little talk" which would follow. The meeting agenda was full of the usual heavy items about budgets, targets and standards. Despite its turgid and demanding timbre, I found myself absorbed and drawn into the complex discussions. This was what I was good at; I worked hard, had prepared well and could hold my own with colleagues who were often competitive and challenging. Whether I was gnawing away at Sam, unable to give in and move on, or working on some project, report or scheme at work, the activity became utterly absorbing. The problem was that in consequence my life contained no sense of balance, no middle ground or still point where I could find real peace in the moment. My obsessions clashed like gladiators on the field of battle, a perpetual struggle which never resulted in victory or defeat, played endlessly within my head. I never allowed myself to stop and consider that the preservation of my sanity might require some resolution, that the strain of such frantic struggle might be causing me real harm.

After the meeting, I just wanted to escape. Despite my interest in the subject matter, throughout I had been aware of a feeling of sickness and despair deep within. I had given myself no time to deal with or reflect on the consequences of my latest engagement with Sam and I knew that the cumulative effect of layer upon layer of rejection and disappointment was pushing me to the limit. I retreated to the toilets, the privacy behind the locked door allowing the first moment of reflection since the morning's stressful events. I caught my breath, realising I was close to tears and wanting to run away, find a place to hide where I might at least allow myself to release the tension and clear my thoughts. Knowing that the journey back to my office would be far less stressful, I became desperate to make my departure, enclose myself in the personal sanctuary of my car.

As I left the cubicle the administrative supervisor, Shirley, came through the door. She asked if we could have a chat about a mutual project. This was the last thing I needed but, caught off guard and weakened by the morning's events, I was unable to extricate myself. Shirley was a smart and confident woman in late middle age, the kind of person for whom life has always proved agreeable. I knew that Shirley had been married for many years to her devoted husband, who picked her up from the office at the end of each day and even made her packed lunch in the mornings. I liked Shirley and at some level envied her steady and peaceful life, but we shared only a business relationship and I felt no personal affinity. We found a quiet corner in the staff room and began to chat. To my horror, I found myself unable to engage or concentrate. On the verge of tears, hoping to avoid embarrassment, I took a deep breath which only served to emphasise my obvious distress. Shirley's simple "what's the matter?" precipitated a fit of desperate and uncontrollable weeping from which there was no retreat.

I had no choice but to surrender to the situation. Having, for so long, made elaborate efforts to hide my mental anguish from those closest to me, ironically I now found myself comforted by someone with whom I had only the most superficial of relationships. My cover was finally broken in the most humiliating way. I felt out of control, weary with the stress of hiding away and making excuses, alone and exposed. I told Shirley a little of the story, just enough to give a rudimentary explanation, then finally able to reassure her that I would be OK and must leave as I had things to do, I drove back to the privacy of my office.

Once behind closed doors, rather than allow myself to crumble and release more pent up emotion, I repaired my makeup and started to go through my post. My secretary put her head around the door and asked if I would like some tea. I had grown to like Julia very much after twelve months of working with her. Although I had never disclosed the details of my unhappiness to Julia, I knew that she had gleaned that something was badly wrong. If there was anyone I could trust with confidences I desperately needed to share it was Julia, yet even the safety of this knowledge had not been enough to enable me to let go. I was simply too ashamed.

I accepted the offer of tea, and Julia asked if all was well. I gave my usual dismissive response, blaming pressure of work and overtiredness for my harassed appearance. Eventually we got back to work. There were several routine messages, some letters to sign and a request from my boss that I ring him. Finally, there was a message which completely took me aback, a request for a return call from my old friend Steve. I had no idea how he had found me, I hadn't heard from him in ten years. My first thought was "what the hell does he want?"

I waited until Julia had left the office then picked up the phone to ring my boss. Jim was a pleasant and approachable man; now promoted to the next level, he was a former colleague who had been my line manager for the last year. After enquiring whether I was OK, Jim suggested that we should meet soon, perhaps over lunch. When I asked what he wanted to discuss, Jim became a little hesitant. Clearly uncomfortable with 'emotional issues', he managed to convey his concern that I seemed distracted and he wanted to find out if there was anything he could do to help. After agreeing a date and ending the conversation, I sat in silence knowing that, despite Jim's tolerant and affable approach, his main concern would be to ensure that the standard of my work wasn't slipping. I had tried so hard to compartmentalise, to preserve the sanctity of the one thing which provided escape and fulfilment in my otherwise barren existence; now even that was threatened with infiltration.

Feeling a sense of desolation and unhappiness which threatened again to reduce me to tears, I spotted the telephone number written on a yellow "post it" note on my desk. Steve. Strangely, despite the fact that I had not seen or heard from Steve for ten years, I had known what Julia was going to say in the split second before she said it. Not so much "old boyfriend" as former colleague, I had worked closely with Steve for three years. Both in long-term relationships at the time, we found ourselves enjoying a clandestine and light-hearted affair which involved frequent sex and a few stolen weekends of fun and giggles. At first, I found myself becoming emotionally attached, but when I realised that Steve had no intention of moving the relationship to another level, I had suppressed my feelings and accepted it for what it was. For all that, our liaison had lasted for three years. It all ended after my first marriage finally fell apart. Steve had remained with his partner, showing no sign of wanting to change that situation. Shortly afterwards, I met Sam.

My contact with Steve had continued in the form of infrequent phone calls, invariably instigated by Steve. Tragically, a few months after I met Sam, Steve's partner, Faye, had died. I was overcome with guilt. Despite Steve's encouragement that we should meet, I refused, regarding my relationship with Sam as worthier and guilt-free. Eventually Steve and I lost touch.

Handling the "post-it" note for a few seconds, I slipped it into my desk drawer and packed up to go home.

As I drove home, the sun was setting over the sea. Land-locked for most of my life, I had always wanted to live on the coast. Whatever my mood, however stressed I felt, I never failed to be grateful for the beautiful surroundings in which I lived. It felt as though life always provided some kind of compensation, a foil to the hostility and loneliness which overshadowed me. Wanting to delay my arrival at home for as long as possible, I headed for the beach.

Sitting in the car, sheltered from the bitterness of the wind and feeling only the peace and calm of the natural environment, I closed my eyes. For a long time, I had abandoned any idea that I might be happy; I seemed only intent on subsuming myself into a different version of the current struggle. All my energy was spent trying to change Sam back into the person I had first met, the charming, attentive and amusing man who had quickly sought security in a new relationship, having recently separated. Knowing I wasn't ready, I had allowed myself to be seduced, quite literally, by the promise of relief from panic at the thought of being left alone. All the danger signs had appeared very early in the relationship, yet I rationalised and persisted. Night thoughts and doubts were banished, attributed to the stress of too much change, and events moved quickly; before I could question my judgement, I had agreed to marry him.

Lately I had begun to meditate, a lonely practice which I learned from self-help literature. Sitting in the warm car, eyes closed, I sensed the glow of the red-shifted light on the horizon, silently begging for help from whatever higher power might be listening. It seemed so little to ask, I didn't want a sense of freedom or a passionate new love, but a miracle which would transform Sam into the person I thought I had met. That morning, once again I had tried so hard to reason with him. Ignoring what I well knew, that our relationship was more like parent and child than an equal partnership, I had pleaded with Sam to take me out for the evening, hoping that the relaxed atmosphere of the local pub or even a restaurant might allow us a rare opportunity to talk about how we might improve our relationship. The response was the same as always, absolutely not! What I also knew, and again ignored, was that my pleading fed Sam's need for power and dominance, allowed him again and again to disappoint and control. Unable to deal rationally with my own needs and simply walk away, I had persisted in driving further and further from me the things I most desired. I wanted so little, just to have some fun, explore together the beautiful place where we lived, bring back a little gentleness and respect for each other. Instead I was left with a relationship stripped of all intimacy, characterised by bitterness and hostility in which I repeated, over and over, my child-like pleading. Like a film constantly being replayed by a fool who somehow thinks that next time the ending will change, the scenario invariably culminated in devastating rejection.

Finally, I opened my eyes and started the car. When I arrived home, late in the evening and laden with shopping, Sam neither acknowledged my arrival nor offered to help me with the bags. His only comment, sometime later, was "what's for tea?" After a long, exhausting and emotional day, I threw together a meal and went to bed. Several hours later, Sam crawled in beside me, barely disturbing my sleep. Despite the long-term absence of a physical relationship, he had refused to consider separate rooms.

Side by side, together through proximity alone, we spent the night in silence.

4.

WEEKEND

"One moves with an uncertain violence
Under the dust thrown by a baffled sense
Or the dull thunder of approximate words"

Thom Gunn, 'On the Move'

Despite all the evidence to the contrary, I always expected that my weekends would provide a pleasant break from weekly routine; I was frequently disappointed.

Sam and I had accumulated a great deal of 'dirty washing', repeat recriminations and tit for tat behaviours prompted by past disappointment, and our individual bids for power within the relationship. I was ashamed of my behaviour at times, yet the only power I felt I could wield was to refuse the things Sam still required of me, to sabotage what mattered most to him. At times the triumph was delicious, yet ultimately, I always lost. I tended to threaten and manipulate where I sensed Sam was vulnerable. His Achilles' heel was his relationship with his daughter, Helen. In a display of what I saw as the most extreme hypocrisy, in Helen's presence Sam would once again turn into an affable and charming person, his hostility gone and in its place the demonstrative and gregarious behaviour I recognised from our early relationship.

When things first began to go badly wrong in our relationship,

Sam had publicly displayed affection towards me in front of others, giving the impression to the outside world that all was well, instantly reverting to cruelty and harshness once we were alone. I had long since made clear to him that I found this utterly unacceptable; we ultimately settled into a sterile routine, where I would escape to the kitchen, leaving Sam to entertain our guests, almost always members of his family or his friends. My friends and relations had backed off incrementally, sensing an atmosphere of hostility and rejection.

This weekend, Helen and her partner Tom were due to visit. As usual I consulted my favourite cookery books, shopped for special ingredients, made the house warm and comfortable. In the hours before Tom and Helen were due to arrive, Sam and I began to bicker. Our mutual hostility rose to a crescendo an hour or so before the young couple were expected. Fuelled by some unresolved past disagreement, the dispute became more and more acrimonious. Finally, I refused to continue preparing the evening meal, accusing Sam of hypocrisy and favoritism, reminding him of the way he had isolated me from the people I loved. I desperately wanted to walk out, to leave him alone with his deception and falsehood exposed to the elements, forcing him to explain to Helen why I was not there, humiliated in front of his daughter as I had so often been humiliated in the presence of those I cared about.

The truth was I liked Helen. In a perverse sort of way I looked forward to her visits, which provided a rare oasis of relief from the monotony of life with Sam. At times Helen had confided in me, intimating that her father's behaviour towards her own mother had been less than acceptable and expressing concern for my welfare. In return, I had confessed to the true nature of my relationship with Sam, knowing that ultimately Helen's loyalty would be towards her father but having no other means of expressing my feelings. At least there was one person who knew first-hand the reality of what I was going through and who could see beyond the facade which Sam so consummately projected to the outside world.

Despite my strong desire to wound Sam in some way I did not walk out on him, I did not leave him to explain himself, nor did I expose his duplicity. For complex reasons I played along with the farcical and dishonest picture he wished to paint. In no way was this an unselfish act; I knew that to withdraw would simply delay the pain and recrimination which would inevitably follow. I also had a desperate need for company and stimulation. For all these reasons I cooked and I served and I stayed out of the way while Sam fawned and performed for his daughter and her partner.

Dinner was ready. I laid the table, served the dishes and for the first time, sat down with our guests. Sam continued to dominate the conversation, impressing Tom with an embellished story about a recent outing. Helen and Tom complimented me on my cooking and hospitality and Helen asked me how my job was going. For many years, Sam had decried, belittled and criticised my career. He had refused to discuss the details of my working life and berated me as narcissistic for discussing my job with friends. Having failed adequately to deal with my feelings about the bitter row with Sam before our guests' arrival, I simply could not play along. The only response I would permit myself was "I'm not allowed to talk about my job." Even in the knowledge that this would later evoke a severe reaction from Sam, I could not bring myself to make some superficial response in order to deflect attention from myself and allow Sam to continue his consummate performance.

The conversation stopped and in the silence all the pain, all the fear, all the suppressed and destructive emotions within me seemed to conspire against my attempts at composure. I began to sob, a shaking, uncontrollable and violent expression of years of negativity. In my accompanying embarrassment, I tried to curtail my emotions, serving only to exacerbate the situation. Incredibly, Sam continued to talk as though nothing had happened, completely ignoring me. Tom, whose relationship with Helen was relatively new, looked confused and desperately uncomfortable, all the more for Sam's bizarre behaviour. Realising that I had little choice, I left the table, retreated to the bedroom and continued to cry.

A little time later, Helen came up to the bedroom. She asked me how I was, then began to talk in the manner of someone revealing secrets, slightly uncomfortable but resolute. "There's something you ought to know. You won't be surprised by what I have to say and I know I've hinted at this before, but I didn't want to say more out of loyalty to my dad. I guess I was hoping that he might have changed. My mum endured many years of abuse from my dad, nothing she did was right. He disliked her friends and family and rubbished her interests, stifled her independence and tried to stop her doing the things she loved. They had no life together, no social life and little contact with friends. When she protested and tried to reason with him, he made her feel that she was wholly responsible for his behaviour, that he would have been different if she had treated him differently. Occasionally he was also physically abusive. I hope he has never hit you, but even if he hasn't I want to warn you that could happen. This is not about you, it's about him." I was touched by her confidences and knew that this was difficult for Helen.

Helen continued, "I know that my dad can change in an instant and that other people don't see his extreme behaviour. This was the most distressing thing for my mother, it made her feel completely alone. Many times, she tried to tell mutual friends about what was happening but she was left with the impression they didn't believe her, he was so different when they were around. Only her personal friends picked up his hostility and she was too embarrassed by his behaviour to confide in them until she had to because she could stand no more. I wanted you to know that I'm not fooled; now I've seen this for myself I can tell you that I saw plenty of distressing behaviour when I was growing up. My dad may be sweetness and light when I'm around, but that's only because there is distance between us now, I'm an independent adult and I've been placed in the category of people he wants to impress. Don't get me wrong, I know he loves me and for all his faults, I love him. I just wanted you to have the whole picture; and I guess I wanted to tell you to protect yourself, get out while you can. You're an attractive, intelligent woman, you deserve better than this."

I was very grateful and lost for words. I began to sob again, and Helen touched my arm: "Just get out! Promise me you'll keep in touch? I want to know what's happening and if I can do anything to help, I will." I agreed, sensing the urgency that Helen needed to go.

As I lay on my back on the bed, staring at the ceiling, it occurred to me that I had spent many hours of my life crying alone in my room. It seemed that, as soon as I began to develop my own ideas or assert myself as an independent being, there had been someone holding me back, violently disagreeing with my views and beliefs and causing me to feel belittled and misunderstood. I felt alone and very sorry for myself. From downstairs came the sounds of animated but pleasant conversation, as though life went on perfectly well without me, despite the considerable efforts I had made to welcome our guests. I was suddenly overcome with a sense of terrible injustice; I could not understand why my life had been so unhappy, why did some people seem to drift along without fear or trauma and others felt such pain? These were precious moments of my one life, never to be experienced again and yet I was spending them alone in a darkening room, full of shadows and sorrow.

After a while, I heard Tom and Helen leaving. Despite Helen's confession, which should have provided me with the objective proof I needed that Sam's behaviour was entrenched and unlikely to change, somewhere inside I still hoped that Sam would come and comfort me, apologise for his oppressive behaviour and put things right. Intellectually, I knew that this was never going to happen. Emotionally, I still harboured an irrational hope that the situation was retrievable.

Sam did not come. I stayed in the darkness of the bedroom, eventually drifting into sleep.

At two am I woke abruptly from a troubled dream. Sam slept beside me, oblivious to my trauma. Events of the day before reassembled themselves in my mind like a tragedy, haunting and hopeless. What was the dream? Half-remembered but powerful images from my subconscious conspired to prevent me from falling back to sleep. In my dream I had been sitting on a bus, driven by my father. The bus was climbing a very steep hill at a slow pace and was full of people, all looking at me and laughing manically. In dream imagery, laughter means tears.

The next day was Sunday. I expected Sam to react badly to me, to chastise and punish. Instead he refused to talk, blanked me when I challenged him to get on with it, hopeful for any reaction and ready for conflict myself. This simply enraged me. I was desperate to express my anger, ready to scream and accuse, demand answers and spend endless hours pushing Sam for a resolution. Instead Sam refused to engage, finding renewed power in denial. He watched TV, mowed the lawn, read the paper. He was clearly enjoying my pain.

5.

Steve

*"Angels come in many shapes and sizes and
most of them are not invisible."*

Martha N. Beck, 'Expecting Adam'

By Monday, I was exhausted. I knew I should have stayed at home but pushed myself to go to work, desperate not to fail at that as well. Delayed again, this time through sheer exhaustion which caused me to sleep late, I dragged myself into the office.

After a morning of e-mails, phone calls and hassle, I went out to meet my manager, Jim, for lunch. I was prepared for the mild telling off I knew was coming, but not for Jim's genuine concern for my welfare. Forced recently to reveal far more than I had intended, I was reluctant to say too much to Jim. When his gentle probing about my 'wellbeing' got too near the knuckle I shrugged it off with some vague comments about feeling off colour and needing a holiday. Jim, who was intensely uncomfortable with personal intrusion, seized on the opportunity to encourage me to take some leave, a concrete and practical solution he could record as an 'outcome' in his note of our meeting. Thus, I was able once again to retreat to the false security of isolation and avoidance; preferable, it seemed, to the humiliation of once more having to expose my sense of embarrassment and personal failure.

The next day Julia, who had somehow sensed more than a business connection in the contact from Steve, tried to press me for more information. I gave a vague response, indicating that we had been friends as well as colleagues. I told her that I wasn't sure I was going to return his call, which was the truth. I didn't feel I had the time and wasn't sure I had the inclination.

By the middle of the week I had regained my composure. A work project was coming together well and I was doing what I did best; bringing people together and inspiring them to solve problems. I loved to make good things happen, knew I was skilled at leadership and well-liked by the staff. In contrast to the negativity and rejection of my personal relationships, when things were good at work my job provided the positive affirmation I so needed.

At times I wondered how I could possibly attract such opposing reactions, doubted my sanity when the space of a day or so could bring praise and reward from my career, tempered with harsh and dismissive invective from Sam, whose main preoccupation was his own needs.

I found myself working late once more, this time out of sheer enthusiasm. Julia had left early, and the office was quiet; I sorted through a large pile of papers, organised my agenda for the next day and cleared my e-mails. I made myself a coffee and sat back in my chair, watching the light fade through the large sash windows. The upstairs room provided a beautiful view of the seaside town. As I watched, the coloured lights along the shore began to glow and I could see the stream of heavy traffic on the coast road. Not for the first time, I wondered where everyone was going and imagined the state of domestic bliss to which the rest of the world returned at the end of a productive day. At moments like these, my sense of realism and perspective retreated. I had become detached from the light and shade of human existence, and my self-image took on the form of a wretched and disgraced outsider, someone who felt she had no respectable role in society. My behaviour was variously superficial and insincere, cowering and hopeless against a world of shining people with perfect relationships.

The triumphs of the day effectively exorcised, I packed up to go home. Home; the concept should have given me pleasure after a good day's work. Home should be safe and welcoming, warm and enticing. In truth, since my adolescence, I had never felt this way about home. Since becoming an adult I had always loved the bricks and mortar, choosing attractive houses and making them comfortable and inviting. In contrast my relationships with men had been destructive and deeply disappointing, failing to complement the physical environment. No matter how bad things had been in the past, though, nothing compared to the desolation of my relationship with Sam.

Suddenly I thought about the telephone number in the drawer. My thoughts turning to Steve I felt a strong urge to speak to my friend. It had been a couple of weeks since he had left the message and I had been unsure about returning his call. I wasn't entirely clear why I hesitated to ring him; had I simply become so isolated that I was out of the habit of speaking to my friends? It had been a long time. I tried to recall his face, failing to bring its substance to mind. What I could remember was the way he made me laugh, the way we had distracted each other from work and the fun we had together. My relationship with Steve had been unlike any other I had ever experienced with a man.

Not expecting a reply, I rang the number. To my surprise he answered, and within seconds the old comfortable familiarity returned, as though we had never been parted. He called me a "silly tart" for not ringing earlier, the characteristic taunting a poignant contrast to my conversations with Sam. Even so, I was very guarded. In response to Steve's curiosity about my relationship with Sam, I was non-committal, not wishing to confess or confide. We caught up a little and teased each other about how we must have changed since we last met. Steve was going to be visiting the south coast within a few weeks and wanted to meet for lunch. Despite my former hesitation, I agreed to the meeting.

Reflecting afterwards on our conversation, I realised how much I had missed Steve's friendship, his persistence and his sense of humour. Well beyond the end of our affair, it was my lack of commitment which had caused our occasional contact to fizzle out.

Steve had continued to ring me at work, wanting to chat and occasionally asking if we could meet, until my refusals and persistent failure to return his calls had discouraged him completely. It would be good to see him again.

6.

RAGE

"To live a life that is wrong for you is a form of dying."

Martha N. Beck, 'Finding Your Own North Star'

Sam did not want to go on holiday. I had always loved holidays abroad, but holidays with Sam had become tortuous and stressful. Finally, he had taken to refusing to consider or plan them, part of his campaign to deny me the things that mattered most. Lacking the confidence to take a holiday on my own or with a friend, I would repeatedly plead with him to give in. He would typically refuse to consider a holiday until late in the year, when it was more difficult to find good weather, then reject my suggestions, finally agreeing to go under his terms. I would do all the work myself to find a holiday to fit his criteria.

I was tired and in need of a break. Long working hours, emotional exhaustion and taking responsibility for managing the household had left me craving sunshine and relaxation. Once again, I tried to get Sam to discuss the prospect of a trip abroad, but he simply refused to entertain the idea. After prolonged pleading, Sam agreed to go if I did all the organising. He insisted on Portugal, which I didn't fancy and where I knew we were unlikely to experience good weather this late in the season. Attempts to get him to consider more favourable climates failed, so I accepted, at least assured of a trip abroad. I booked the trip; we would be leaving in two weeks' time.

I rarely spent evenings out with friends. A week before the holiday, I planned to meet Julia for dinner in town, my first evening outing in more than a year. Sam was not happy. He grumbled about having to get his own dinner and expressed his disapproval of my outfit, finally sending me through the door with an insulting comment about my appearance. Utterly defeated by his selfishness and negativity, and now no longer in the mood for a night out, I set off to meet my friend.

Julia was a strong and independent young woman. She lived alone, her last relationship having ended in acrimony some time before. She had little trust in men and enjoyed her self-sufficiency. Over our meal, we gossiped about life at the office, putting the world to rights.

Eventually we turned to more personal matters. I teased Julia about an admirer who regularly pursued her and whose advances she steadfastly rejected and found myself laughing uncontrollably. It had been so long since I had enjoyed myself like this.

The conversation somehow turned to my personal affairs and Julia enquired after my welfare. I was immediately on my guard and asked Julia if Shirley had confided in her. Realising that I had now implied that all was not well, I took a deep breath and confessed. I found myself confiding in Julia about the hostility, the conflict and the abuse. This time it was a relief to talk. I really did trust Julia and enjoyed her companionship both as a colleague and a friend. Julia was horrified. "He would only have to hit me once and I'd be gone, why ever do you stay?" Stopped short by the starkness of the question, I sat back and reflected. I explained that people underestimate the complexity of such situations, that it was my home as much as Sam's and that he used to be so kind. Even to myself, however, the explanation sounded feeble. However complex the situation might have been, the answer should have been simple. "Forgive me, but it doesn't sound like he's very kind now," said Julia. That was as much as I could take. I diverted the conversation and suggested it was time to go home.

As I drove through the dark streets, I felt a growing sense of emotional discomfort. I had hidden my problems with Sam for so long, without a whisper to the outside world, yet in a short space of time I had endured the exposure of my innermost feelings to a colleague with whom I had little affinity, attracted the attention of my boss for the wrong reasons, lost my composure in front of Helen and found myself confiding in Julia, resulting in her inevitable probing. Whilst the enclosure of my former isolation had brought little comfort, it had become familiar and somehow engendered a false sense of safety; within its confinement I could protect myself from facing the enormity of my problems and the pain of revelation. I began to recognise that the more my secrets were revealed, the more I felt an obligation to demonstrate that I could overcome this situation. Failure to do so would, at best, cause embarrassment and make me appear weak; at worst it would confirm to the outside world that I was a failure, different and less worthy than those around me.

I was hoping that Sam would be in bed. Seeing the lights from the house as I pulled up the drive, I began to feel apprehensive. Lately, Sam's presence had become even more threatening. I had occasionally found myself startled when he arrived home, my stomach churning with dread. I opened the door quietly, hoping that he had simply left the lights on for me, but Sam was in the hall, his immediate "Where the hell have you been?" stunning me at first. "I've been out with Julia, you know that, where do you think I've been?"

"Look at the time, a grown woman staying out until now."

I could take no more, screaming, "Oh, fuck you!" I tried to push past him and mount the stairs.

He caught me by the hair, dragging me back down. I became enraged and frightened all at once; all I wanted to do was go to bed alone. I managed to pull away and ran up to the bedroom, trying to close the door and drag a cupboard behind it. Sam was too quick; he caught up with me, shoved me on to the bed and put his hands around my throat, banging my head against the pillow again and again. Finally, Sam stopped, leaving me sobbing into the pillow, desperate and afraid. I screamed at him to leave me alone. Mercifully, he retreated to the spare bedroom.

A few hours of darkness and sleeplessness later, I heard a wailing sound coming from the landing outside my bedroom door. Crouched in the corner, Sam was in foetal position and crying like a small child, begging my forgiveness. Exhausted with fear and lack of sleep, I let him into my bed. I lay awake until first light, my back to Sam, his arms clinging tightly around my waist.

From early in our relationship, I had known that Sam was suffering from a mental imbalance; his childlike demands for immediate attention, obsession with his health and frequent aggression were not the actions of a rational person. Yet his ability to control and alter his behaviour in an instant in the company of others betrayed a more calculating aspect to his personality, and an indication of a more sinister intent.

I told no-one about the violent incident which followed my night out with Julia. For many years I had felt ashamed of my failed relationships. Surrounded by family and friends who tended to have long-term, stable partnerships, at least they seemed so, I felt inadequate and unworthy. My approach to the problems with Sam was to try and seek help to put Sam's problems right. Sam's refusal to consider joint counselling or support left me grasping for remedies from other sources. His constant obsession with his health problems, many of them imagined, had left me exasperated. He would frequently expect me to show sympathy and understanding but refuse to seek medical help. When he became sufficiently convinced that he was desperately ill, he would eventually visit his doctor, invariably resulting in a series of tests, most of which would prove clear.

After his attack on me, Sam took to bed for several days. His regret did not last long and I would arrive home from work to find that he had done nothing to help in the house, no meal was prepared and he would still be wearing his pyjamas. He would complain of aches and pains, convinced that he was having a heart attack, hold his head in his hands and berate me for showing no sympathy. I had no idea what to do and my pleas that he visit the doctor were met with vitriol.

I finally contacted the doctor myself. This was not the first time and the conversation always started the same way. I would explain why I was there, I would be told that the doctor could not discuss confidential information and I would explain that I simply wanted to convey information, not receive it, in the hope that it would provide a background which would enable the right referral to be made, should Sam visit the surgery himself. Instead of realising that my efforts to change Sam's behaviour   were in vain I lived constantly in the hope that someone could help, someone could save the hopeless and desperate situation in which I found myself, maybe with a referral to the right source or simply the right words. On these visits, I never gave away the full the extent of the abuse I was suffering, concentrating on Sam's "problems."

My efforts, as usual, were in vain; Sam refused to visit the doctor. Even more distressing, two days before our holiday, Sam decided that he was not going. I felt as though I was falling apart. I was so desperate for a holiday, craving the warmth and relaxation, even imagining that Sam would be different if I could persuade him to relax.

Having taken a couple of days leave to prepare for the holiday, I could not bear to remain in the house with Sam. Again, I retreated to the sea. It was one of those not infrequent moments in my life when I literally had no idea what to do. I suspected that Sam was just playing games, but I had no idea how to respond. Against the evidence, I was always hopeful that our holidays would provide the sense of retreat and excitement I so badly needed. I wanted to go. I wanted to enjoy my holiday. Incredibly, I wanted Sam to go with me.

It was a chilly day in early autumn. The beach was storm-blown and beautiful; white breakers and crashing waves. Few people were out and about, but I watched as a group ran along the beach trailing a kite, a small dog in pursuit, barking with joy. A family, people who loved each other and were happy enough to plan a joint trip to the beach, even to enjoy a game together. So distant from the world I inhabited, they looked like aliens from another planet. Somehow I couldn't quite believe they were real. I felt a familiar sensation, like I was in a goldfish bowl, looking out on a distorted and unfamiliar world, utterly alone and distanced from reality. Everyone else seemed happy, or at least in control; I was neither, and saw no hope of redemption. This was a sense of loneliness so profound it was almost comforting and poetic, like Keats's 'drowsy numbness', which dulled the senses and brought blissful relief from harshness and cruelty.

Shaking myself, I decided to ring Julia, this time I had to tell someone. Julia's reaction was genuine, the authentic compassion of a true friend. She didn't know what to say or do, but it didn't matter, I needed simply to express my sense of hopelessness. "I'm supposed to be going on holiday the day after tomorrow and I have no idea whether that's going to happen. Do I pack? Do I try to cancel? I suspect he will come along in the end, but do I really want that?"

At the end of the conversation, I was left again with the prospect of returning to Sam. He was still in the chair where I had left him, watching TV and ignoring my return. I decided once again to try and reason with him and get some clarity about what we were going to do. Of course, it was futile. He refused to commit himself; I realised that he took great pleasure in the pain this caused, reinforcing his sense of absolute power. I felt unable either to control the situation or to make decisions. I packed our case, knowing that he was likely to relent at the last moment and, incredibly, still desperate for us both to go.

With time on my hands, I began to sort through a pile of books I was thinking of sending to a charity shop. There were many books in my house. Having loved to read from a very early age, I could never bear to part with them, believing that they would somehow provide me with insight and inspiration just when it was needed. I came across an old Bible. I had no idea it was there. I had not practised conventional religion since my childhood, yet I felt a strong spiritual connection and awareness which sometimes provided inexplicable and miraculous experience. With a sense of desperation and hoping for some comfort, I opened pages at random, but nothing struck me as significant. I was about to put the Bible back when it fell open at the first page. There was an inscription in my father's handwriting, "I can do all things through Christ which strengtheneth me," a quote from a religious convention he had attended.

Moved to tears, I recalled the father of my early childhood, his wisdom and gentleness, humour and kindness. As a child, I had thought he knew everything, trusted him implicitly. Many times, in his presence, I would close my eyes, knowing that even in a state of sensory deprivation I was completely safe with him. Suddenly I missed the dad who loved me so much, who protected and cared for me in the midst of a confusing and sometimes hostile family environment. I knew I had been searching for him all my adult life. The intimacy which was lost when I became a wilful and independent teenager devastated me and generated a period of conflict which seemed to go on forever, spilling over again and again as my subsequent relationships, initially so hopeful, began repeatedly to fail.

I knew that, in all my arguments and disputes with Sam, and before him with my first husband, Joe, I was simply replaying my attempts to reach my father, repeating the futile pattern of struggle and despair. Then, like now, the act of attempting to change someone else in order to find my own happiness was pointless and utterly destructive, yet I could not seem to break away. I understood the theory and knew that I was locked into a futile life pattern, giving in to excess in the hope of putting things right instead of walking away from situations which other people would not tolerate. This had nothing to do with love. I had ceased to love Sam a long time ago and often yearned desperately to be free.

The Eagles encapsulated exactly how I felt, in their beautiful song, "Wasted Time":

"The autumn leaves have got you thinking, about the first time that you fell,

You didn't love the boy too much, no, you just loved the boy too well."

Astounded by the message from my father, just when I was feeling so desolate, I took the Bible and placed it by my bed.

7.

HOLIDAY

*"I have allowed myself to lead this little life when
inside me there was so much more. And it's all gone
unused. And now it never will be. Why do we get
all this life if we don't ever use it? Why do we get
all these feelings and dreams and hopes
if we don't ever use them?"*

Willy Russell, 'Shirley Valentine'

Two days later, we were on our way to Portugal. Sam had prolonged the agony until the last minute, ultimately feigning grudging capitulation. I had been furious, despite my prediction that this was going to happen, and our last-minute preparations had been fraught and ill-humoured.

It was not a pleasant journey; we drove to the airport in silence, queuing at the check in desk side by side, but looking anywhere except at each other. We could not get seats together on the plane. I sat in an aisle seat two rows back from Sam, headphones providing a welcome detachment from the world around me. Beautiful music overwhelming my senses, tears began to pour down my cheeks. I was horrified to notice that the passenger next to me was watching me cry, turning away swiftly when I caught him looking. Had I been sobbing out loud?

45

Portugal was chilly, with long, dark evenings. I had tried to warn Sam that the Atlantic coast was dodgy at this time of year, but he insisted that the weather would be fine as someone he knew had recommended it. He would habitually ignore my ideas and suggestions, giving precedence to the views and opinions of strangers and casual acquaintances. We had hired a villa with a pool, which we hardly used due to the chill in the air. Sam was unbelievably obstructive and negative; at times his behaviour was bizarre. He knew that I loved to eat out, trying different restaurants and being waited on for once. Each evening he would go and lie on the bed around six, protesting that he couldn't be bothered to change and go out. I would get changed for dinner, not daring to disturb him in case he refused to come with me. Sometimes he would emerge ready to go out but grudging and abusive, other times he would simply refuse to leave and I would find myself making a meal with the basic and unpalatable ingredients from the fridge, in a dark and unwelcoming kitchen designed as a functional room to support sunlit nights on the terrace.

Days were not much better. I disliked the part of the Algarve we had chosen. The scenery was bleak, the beaches featureless. Sam now believed, without substantiation, that he had a serious heart complaint. He would throw himself into violent coughing fits and clutch desperately at his chest. During one outing he was driving along a busy dual carriageway when, without warning, he flung open the car door and began to cough violently, almost making himself sick while the car continued to roll along. I was petrified, my panicky reaction making no impact on Sam, who simply became more aggressive.

It was a relief to get home. I knew I needed to do something, but in my tortured and distorted mind I could not see the simple truth, that I just had to walk away.

The day before I was due back at work was the day on which I had agreed to meet Steve. It wasn't easy to get away from Sam; when I was at home, he watched my movements closely, often blocking in my car with his and refusing to move it to let me go out. After the inevitable interrogation about where I was going, I managed to get away, making some excuse about having to call into the office. The sense of freedom as I drove along was profound. I realised that I had absolutely no expectations of this meeting; in fact I had given it very little thought. I was simply going to meet an old friend who used to make me smile.

We had agreed to meet in a small cove with a coffee bar. I parked my car, emerging to smell the sea air. There was a tap on my right shoulder; turning around I saw no one. I turned in the opposite direction just in time to catch a glimpse of blue denim, darting the other way. There was Steve, instantly recognisable and wearing a jacket I knew well. Immediately time contracted. Ten years became ten seconds, the familiar giggle, the child-like behaviour, the sense of freedom and safety returned.

"Give us a kiss!"

"Get off, you silly sod, I'm spoken for."

"Let's go to the coffee bar, I'm dying for a cake."

Instantly we had created an alternative reality which provided more warmth, more fun and more affirmation than I had experienced with Sam in many years.

Driving back home, I reflected on the meeting. Steve was thinner, his hair almost grey, but essentially the same Steve I remembered. The conversation had been light, neither of us directly mentioned our affair, yet we had managed to talk about old times without awkwardness. I discovered that Steve's recollection of some events differed slightly from mine and that some things I remembered with great clarity, he seemed to have forgotten.

We talked only superficially about the events of the past ten years since we had last been in contact. Steve was in a relationship which sounded failing and unhappy. He probed a little about Sam and enquired whether I was happy, to which I simply replied, "I'm not sure life is about happiness."

We had coffee and cake in the small cafe on the shore then walked along the beach a short distance. I found myself becoming anxious after a couple of hours, distracted by the thought of the way Sam would react if I was late back, and wanting to get away. Before we parted, we sat in my car for a few minutes at Steve's insistence, watching the sea. Steve had said "There's a spider on your jumper, perhaps he's called lucky"; simultaneously we proclaimed "spiders are nice", giggling together at the synchronicity.

To my surprise and mild embarrassment, just as he was about to leave the car, Steve threw his arms around me and kissed my hair. I found myself glancing around to make sure no one had seen. He asked if he could ring occasionally and I agreed, though not sure why.

I asked myself what I felt about the encounter. Strangely, the answer was "very little." It was good to see an old friend, nice to escape for a while, but nothing more. Our past relationship had been light but not superficial, a strange combination and unique in my life. It was the only time I could recall having had a physical relationship with a man who was also a good friend. Unencumbered by the pros and cons of emotional commitment, we had been free from baggage and recrimination. When the affair ended, I had simply accepted that it was natural progression, yet I had often thought of him, imagined I would someday meet him in the street and he might not recognise me with short hair.

Now, once again, all I could concentrate on was Sam. Would he somehow sense I had spent time with another man? I drove home faster than I should have, breathless with concern at the thought of more conflict.

Mercifully, when I arrived home all that awaited me was a dark and empty house. Sam had apparently been called by a friend from the golf club and gone out. Thankful and relieved, I made myself some dinner and went to bed to read my book.

9.

REGATTA

"We are all like the bright moon,
we still have our darker side."

Kahlil Gibran, 'The Prophet'

The weekend arrived once more. This time I actually had something to look forward to; it was regatta weekend in a local resort and some of Sam's friends had invited us to meet for lunch on Sunday. Sam went to the golf club weekly, during the day when I was at work. We rarely met with his friends, but on the few occasions we had done so I had enjoyed the outing. Grateful for any social contact and looking forward to having dinner cooked for me, I was glad when Sunday came.

The resort was popular, especially during regatta weekend. As soon as we approached the outskirts of the town, it was clear that parking was not going to be easy. Sam's irritation began as soon as he saw the queues of traffic; having failed to make progress for a few minutes, he began to swear and become abusive. Knowing well that Sam's irritation towards the outside world quickly tended to turn against me, at first I remained silent. Sam did a three-point turn, wheels screeching against the tarmac. He drove too quickly along country lanes, arriving at a parking spot in a remote location, high on a hill above the town. Sam had often used this spot to park, today there were no spaces. I could resist no longer.

"Sam, why don't you try the park and ride?"

His reply was typical, "Keep out of this, I can't believe these bloody people infiltrate the place, we're locals and I'm not paying to park."

Sam drove around for another half hour, still unable to find a space. His anger and frustration reached boiling point, now wholly directed at me; I pleaded with him to take my advice. Finally, not able to accept that his usual parking spot was taken by outsiders, Sam drove back there, becoming almost incoherent with rage that it was still unavailable to him. Beside myself with frustration and anxiety, I could take no more. Opening the car door and grabbing my bag, I yelled, "I'm out of here!" With absolute determination to get away, I began to walk down the hill. I didn't know where I was going and didn't care if I never went home. I just needed to get away.

A minute later, I heard the incessant blaring of a horn and someone shouting. Turning around, I saw Sam's car coming towards me very quickly down the pavement, his head out of the window screaming, "Get in the fucking car!" Shocked into immobility, I stood still as the car approached, coming to a stop inches away from me. Sam threw himself out of the car, grabbed me roughly by the shoulder and pushed me violently through the passenger door. Breathless with fear and shock, I could not even cry. Sam began to drive away again and as he did so I began to sob, pleading for him to let me go and incredulous that even Sam's behaviour could have become so extreme.

Mercifully Sam somehow eventually found a place to park the car. He put his head in his hands and began to wail, begging my forgiveness. We sat in the car for a long time, shaking and sobbing with violent emotion. I would not let Sam touch me, but I made no further bid to escape. I knew that Sam's 'apology' was prompted only by his desperate need not to lose face with his friends, that he only wanted me to accompany him to keep up appearances. Sam wasn't crying because he had upset me, but because he was frustrated and sorry for himself. Incredibly, I found myself trying to calm down and agreeing to go to lunch with him.

Arriving at the lunch venue, Sam entertained his friends with a dramatic and fabricated story, contrived to explain our late arrival. I sat through the meal withdrawn and unresponsive, no doubt leaving the strong impression that the outgoing and gregarious Sam was ill-matched with such a miserable partner.

We did not speak on the journey home. Now that Sam's mission to meet with his friends was accomplished, he showed no sign of wanting to resume his former act of contrition. I went to bed very early. Lying under the covers, curled tightly for security, I replayed the events of the day. I was no fool; I knew I had to leave, to save myself, to bring into the light of day the bright and self-respecting woman I ought to be.

I asked myself what was wrong with me, how could I have so little regard for myself that I subjected myself to such torture? It was nothing short of a miracle that Sam's behaviour had not been witnessed. I imagined with a sense of horror and humiliation the publicity such an event would have attracted, especially as I was now well known in the community through media appearances and interviews.

Where was my sense of balance? I saw myself trapped in Sam's gravity well, like the moon in captured rotation around the earth, able only to show one face, its dark side repressed and unknowable. I had so much to give and deserved so much more. This time I cried only gentle, prolific tears, my body too exhausted even to sob. I drifted off to sleep, my only escape from fatigue and loneliness.

10.

OLD FRIEND

*"I held your hand through all of these years,
you still have all of me."*

Evanescence, 'My Immortal'

On Monday, I went to work as usual. During the management meeting, to which I arrived ten minutes late, my mobile phone, which I had forgotten to turn off, began to ring. Dazed and disorientated, instead of apologising for the intrusion and turning the phone off, I stumbled from the room answering the call as I did so. It was Steve.

"Why aren't you returning my phone calls?"

"I can't speak now, I'm in a meeting."

Steve had left several messages, asking me to ring him, all of which I had ignored. He had even contacted Julia a couple of times hoping to speak to me, the two of them becoming very friendly and chatty. Desperate to get back to the meeting I said.

"Look, ring me tomorrow after 2pm."

"Will you take my call?" Steve asked.

"Yes, I promise," anything to get away and try to retrieve the situation.

Returning to my office the next day I was confronted by a determined Julia.

"Sit there and I'll make you some tea."

"I'm sorry, Julia, I just haven't got time, you know how much work I have to do."

"All the same, I'm making the tea."

I sighed and gave in.

"Steve called, he says you promised to speak to him."

"I know I did, I just can't handle any more demands on my life at the moment. What does he want anyway?"

"He says he's coming down here again in a couple of weeks and he just wants to take you to lunch."

"I have no time, I can't do lunch."

Julia sat back in her chair and gazed at me.

"If you don't mind some feedback, and even if you do, I'm going to give it to you; you never stop, it's like you're running away from yourself, the more you pack into your life, the less time you have to take responsibility for sorting it out. Steve sounds like a nice guy and he just wants to meet for lunch."

I paused for a few seconds,

"I know you're right Julia, but I just can't get to the solution. Starting some kind of liaison with someone else isn't the answer; anyway, Steve isn't the kind of man who makes a lifetime commitment, even if I fancied him and I don't. I'm not even close to sorting out things at home, I can't bear to go home to Sam, so I spend all the time I can at work, even at weekends I lock myself in my office working and we just ignore each other."

"I bet you still cook his meals," said Julia. I said nothing.

"Anyway, I think you should ring Steve back out of courtesy, I'm really not pushing you to start 'something' with him; who am I to advise you on that? I just think you should cultivate your friends, I suspect that's what you need right now."

I did not immediately phone Steve. When Julia left the office, I made some work phone calls and got stuck in to my emails. There was one from Steve, who must have been given the office email address by Julia; for goodness sake, what were they playing at? It was entitled 'The colour of my underpants' and contained a very funny limerick about unrequited love. Despite my mild annoyance, I couldn't contain the giggles, what a fool, he would never grow up. At last I relented and rang his number.

"Ah, 'tis the east and Juliet is the sun, arise, fair sun and kill the envious moon..."

"You'll get me the sack if the IT police do a sweep for personal e mails, you've hardly been subtle."

"Why spoil my reputation now. Anyway, got your attention didn't I?"

Without hesitation we were back into the easy and therapeutic banter of mutually affectionate old friends. Steve wanted to book a train ticket to come and meet me in a couple of weeks; despite myself I relented and put the date in my diary. Characteristically, Steve tried to push the limits.

"...erm, can you get the day off?"

"Absolutely not, that's all you're getting."

The phone call ended, I sat at my desk for a couple of hours tidying up and writing a report. Finally, I had no choice but to leave the office and make my way back to the dark side of the moon.

On the day of my scheduled meeting with Steve the phone never stopped ringing. Normally, Julia and I would have worked through our lunch break to get things completed. Frustrated and harassed, I became resentful about the distraction of having to meet Steve. Finally, as it became clear that I was going to be late, Julia intruded to prompt me to leave. I snatched my handbag and swept out of the door, not at all in the mood for this.

I had agreed to pick Steve up at the station. He was waiting outside, and I drew up beside him, flinging open the passenger door. "Late, I see, fair Juliet." I made a face and he kissed me lightly on the cheek.

We went to another beach. Steve shared my great love of the sea. One of our stolen weekends had been spent in a beautiful and remote part of the mid-Wales coast. I had often thought about that weekend, the isolation and intimacy of a secret retreat about which I had told no one. We ate lunch in a thatched inn and walked along the beach. I had given in and agreed to take the afternoon off, and despite my reticence I began to relax. It felt so good to be free if only for a couple of hours.

We sat on a rock overlooking the sea, laughing and teasing each other. Steve again tried to ask about the nature of my relationship with Sam, but I wouldn't let him in, he wasn't entitled to that information.

He made some comment about the obvious demands of my job and asked where I got my support; another, subtler, means of seeking information. For a few seconds, taken completely by surprise, I simply could not answer. In the end, I just shook my head.

He asked if I was happy with my life and I said that I really couldn't tell him, it was like part of me was missing, I wasn't the person he used to know, the words choking in my throat. Steve touched my hand then gently placed his arm around my shoulders.

"Come on, let's walk to the top of the cliff and get some coffee." On the way up, he asked if we could hold hands. I stopped and turned to him,

"Look, Steve, it's good to see you, but I don't know what you want and I'm not ready for this." He told me, "I want to know more about where you've been, what you've done, how you feel."

I asked him why.

He said. "I think you're a lovely person, I think we have lots in common and I fancy you!"

I punched him on the arm and called him an idiot. We walked to the tea room.

Over coffee we continued to discuss our mutual past, catching up on news of old friends and colleagues. I began once again to become anxious, sensing it was time to leave for home; I still had to call at the supermarket for something for dinner.

As we left the tea room I said, "Well, you've cheered me up, anyway, I never thought anyone would fancy me again!"

Steve stopped and turned to me, gripping my shoulders. "What's the matter with you, I couldn't believe how good you looked when we last met, apart from your hair and a few crow's feet you look exactly the same! Where has your self-confidence gone? You're jumpy and nervous and you never seem to relax." He kissed me on the cheek again and I grinned.

When we reached the station, Steve wanted to talk in the car before he left for the train. I was by now extremely anxious about getting home without risking interrogation or challenge but tried to humour him.

He asked, "Can we meet again, do you ever get away for longer?" I needed to go and said the first thing that came into my head.

"I'm going on a residential course in a month or so, I'll have to stay away the night before- we could meet then." Steve was keen to seize the opportunity.

"OK, I'll ring or email and we can make arrangements." Again, he put his arms around me, this time kissing me on the forehead. By now I just wanted to go and with relief I watched him walk towards the platform, waving as I drove away.

What had I said? How could I get out of this? I liked Steve and was insightful enough to realise that we had an affinity, but I couldn't handle any more complications. Besides, I had made a decision to be faithful to Sam. Exhausted by the strain of my previous relationship which had ended when my partner had confessed to a long affair, about which I could hardly be too judgemental, I had wanted my relationship with Sam to be guilt-free. I was sick of tangled webs. I would have to ring Steve and put him off.

11

AWAKENING

"Cast me gently into morning,
for the night has been unkind."

Sarah Mclachlan, 'Answer'

Sam had been to the golf club and could easily have called for some shopping or a take-away en route home but I knew that he would never offer to do so. I was expected to perform the domestic tasks, which I did without question to prevent even more conflict. Our acrimonious and accusatory arguments left a trail of bitterness so deep it infiltrated our every interaction. For Sam's part, it had obviated any hint of a gesture of goodwill, leaving me with the lion's share of responsibility for managing and financing the practicalities of our life together. Whilst I carried on trying to get Sam to reason and to change, Sam had inferred that I could not provide him with the understanding he demanded. His wants were limitless, his recriminations frequent and his punitive responses to my inability to fill his endless void of need, cruel and heartless. I seemed unable to recognise that no one could ever meet Sam's needs. The harder I tried, the more, in his estimation, I demonstrated my incompetence, and the endless cycle of co-dependence was perpetuated.

That evening, as on many others, apart from the inevitable "What's for tea" from Sam, we did not communicate. Again, I went early to bed to read my book.

At 2am, I found myself jolted awake by my own sobbing. The bed shook with my uncontrollable outpouring, Sam did not stir. I eventually took a blanket and went to sit by the fire in the lounge. It felt like years of suppressed emotions were rising up to attack me, quite literally like a physical assault. What had I done to myself? I had locked myself away with a man who desired only to undermine and destroy me, who was incapable of love and respect for his partner and who took from me daily without guilt or compassion.

I had told myself that life was not about happiness and somehow believed that I must accept my situation without question. In the light of this new insight, I could find no reason why I should have done this, except to suspect that I had made my intention to be faithful to Sam my raison d'etre, even though it now made no sense, and he certainly had not earned my loyalty.

I thought about Steve; lovely, funny, gentle Steve. I remembered things I had buried somewhere in my memory, things which I had put aside because of my initial belief that Sam was the love of my life. I recalled my total obsession with the sense of being in love, which I now knew was a fabrication born of my own desperate need for affirmation. I remembered one of the last phone calls Steve and I had shared before we lost contact; he had said, "I had a friend who used to ring me, I wonder where she went?" The memory of that comment now took my breath away, where *had* I gone? I remembered Steve's frequent suggestions that we should meet, all rejected in favour of Sam and my intention to be honourable. How could I have rejected my friend? I also knew that Steve's careful and deliberate determination to make our romantic association an adjunct to our friendship, and nothing deeper, was a contributory factor. Not once had he given the slightest indication that he wanted anything more.

Needing something to calm me, I decided to play some music on my headphones. All my life, I had found solace and comfort in music, another passion I shared with Steve; and yet another of my pleasures denied by Sam. He would not tolerate my music being played in the house, even to the extent of turning off my stereo without acknowledgment or permission, because it was getting on his nerves or disturbing the TV.

I knew without question what I wanted to play, Eva Cassidy's version of "Time After Time":

> *Lying in my bed I hear the clock tick and think of you,*
> *Turning in circles, confusion is nothing new,*
> *Flash back to warm nights, almost left behind,*
> *A suitcase of memories, time after time*

The words were so apt they touched me at the deepest level. The tears came even faster until I thought they would never stop. Finally, I fell asleep, waking when it was light to find Sam standing over me demanding "Aren't you going to work?"

12.

FIRST STEPS

"The ...far less common meaning of happiness is 'living a rich, full and meaningful life.' When we take action on the things that truly matter deep in our hearts, move in directions that we consider valuable and worthy, clarify what we stand for in life and act accordingly, then our lives become meaningful and we experience a powerful sense of vitality. This is not some fleeting feeling but the sense of a life well lived. And although such a life will undoubtedly give us many pleasurable feelings, it will also give us uncomfortable ones, such as sadness, fear and anger. This is only to be expected, if we live a full life, we will feel the full range of human emotions."

Russ Harris, 'The Happiness Trap'

I knew exactly what I needed to do, but it was very hard. I had a mentor, Liz, who ran a thriving personal training company. Liz and I had worked together for several years, primarily focusing on my job, although she had often tried to probe deeper, sensing that all was not well with my personal life. I had told her I wasn't ready to talk about that.

It would be incredibly difficult to confess to Liz, but I knew that I needed her wisdom and support. With a sense of nervousness born of years of coping alone with my desperate situation, I picked up the phone; I simply said that I needed to talk. Liz's response was decisive and unhesitating, as I knew it would be. We arranged to meet the following week.

Liz and I met at an old abbey part way between our two homes. The setting was peaceful and in the grounds was a restaurant with secluded tables and comfy sofas. We could spend the day there in peace and without fear of interruption.

After an initial coffee, over which I said very little, we decided to walk in the beautiful wooded countryside surrounding the abbey. I knew I simply had to tell it like it was; I began to talk, describing years of formerly undisclosed sub-text to the main plot of my life with Sam, with which Liz was familiar. I described the early warnings which I had rationalised away, the aggression, the hostility, the gradual withdrawal of all pleasure and enjoyment, the growing isolation from the outside world. I described Sam's deliberate refusal to engage in anything I enjoyed, and his disapproval of my job, my friends and my family; I told Liz that he never took me out, criticised my clothes and appearance, would not even go shopping with me for essentials. I recounted a series of violent and threatening incidents, described Sam's unreasonable demands and his obsession with his health, his refusal to seek help and his endless demands for sympathy and understanding which I did not know how to give.

I also described the way my own behaviour had become resentful and stubborn, angry and pleading. I told of my need to find any means to exert power within the relationship which resulted in bitter disputes and acrimony. I described my attempts to make an impact on Sam by refusing the things he cared about and my frequent tendency to capitulate and lose the battle. I described my failed attempts to get help through contact with the medical profession and my growing depression. Finally, I described the recent incidents at work where the cracks were beginning to show and culminated with a description of Sam driving the car towards me down the pavement when we went to the regatta.

Exhausted with the effort but high with a sense of relief at having finally told someone the whole story, I had no perspective on the true horror of the picture I had just painted, nor of the inherent danger which I had so graphically described. Liz had listened in silence. We decided a break in tension was required and went to the restaurant for a sandwich.

After lunch, we found a sofa by the window in a quiet corner. It was late autumn and few people were around; through the window, the magnificent forest was burnished and golden, backlit by gentle sunlight and utterly silent. Gradually, the adrenaline rush stimulated by my outpouring began to subside; supported absolutely by the safety of Liz's deliberate silence, I stared through the window, watching the forest, hypnotised by its warmth and beauty. I began quietly to weep. Knowing that this would come, Liz was there, gentle arms around my shoulders, neither of us needing or wanting to speak.

We sat there for a long time. I felt like my whole life rested in Liz's hands, yet knew that in reality it had always been up to me. Finally, Liz spoke. "You don't need me to tell you what you've just described, or what you need to do. You came here today because you had already worked that out. I am with you, I was always there and you only had to ask. Whatever you need and whenever you need it, I will be there, day or night. The only thing I feel I can do now is to tell you that I don't think you have really grasped how much danger you are in. Sam is not capable of loving you and your constant efforts to drag out of him something he isn't able to give may mean that he will cause you some great harm. Only Sam is responsible for his behaviour, you cannot change him, and you cannot save him. I want you to know that there is always help and there is always another way. I also know that none of this is easy, but you have to walk away, and you have to do it quickly."

I knew the absolute truth of Liz's words, as though some how they had come from within me. She reminded me to re-read Robin Norwood's book, 'Women Who Love too Much'.

I nodded and could say no more. Before we left, we went for one last walk in the forest. Liz led me to a clearing with a wooden seat; as we sat side by side, I produced the Bible I had found with an inscription in my father's handwriting. Liz knew my story, the tale of a damaged childhood and the loss of my father. She knew how precious this message was to me.

Liz handled the Bible, gently turning the pages until she found what she wanted. She said, "Look where it has fallen open now." Under the sunlit trees, Liz began to recite an extract from Paul's first letter to the Corinthians:

"I may speak in tongues of men or of angels, but if I am without love I am a sounding gong or a clanging cymbal. I may have the gift of prophecy and know every hidden truth; I may have faith strong enough to move mountains; but if I have no love, I am nothing. I may dole out all I possess, or even give my body to be burnt, but if I have no love, I am none the better.

Love is patient; love is kind and envies no one. Love is never boastful, nor conceited, nor rude; never selfish, not quick to take offence. Love keeps no score of wrongs, does not gloat over other men's sins, but delights in the truth. There is nothing love cannot face; there is no limit to its faith, its hope, and its endurance.

Love will never come to an end. Are there prophets? Their work will be over. Are there tongues of ecstasy? They will cease. Is there knowledge? It will vanish away; for our knowledge and our prophecy alike are partial, and the partial vanishes when wholeness comes. When I was a child, my speech, my outlook, and my thoughts were all childish. When I grew up, I had finished with childish things. Now we see only puzzling reflections in a mirror, but then we shall see face to face. My knowledge now is partial; then it will be whole, like God's knowledge of me. In a word, there are three things that last forever: faith, hope and love, but the greatest of them all is love."

I couldn't speak. Of all the tears I had shed in the past few weeks, the ones that now fell were the most prolific. How could I have failed so miserably to see the truth?

13.

REASONING

"He may never change. You must stop trying to make him. And you must learn to be happy anyway."

Robin Norwood, 'Women Who Love Too Much'

I decided to try to bring our relationship to an end by attempting to reach an amicable agreement with Sam. On Sunday morning I made coffee and asked if we could talk. So many times, I had tried to reason with Sam, so many hours of trying to get him to make agreements, improve things just a little and restore the relationship we had lost. Sometimes Sam would simply refuse to talk, and we spent days in silence, ignoring each other and living around our sterile routine. At other times he would tolerate these intense discussions, which tended to follow a familiar pattern. I would raise a series of issues, Sam would either be non-committal or unresponsive, which I would take as a hopeful sign, or he would refuse to entertain my suggestions and the discussion would degenerate into an acrimonious argument. I seemed to have an endless capacity for these sessions, suffering from a peculiar and specific form of amnesia which caused me to forget that, time and time again, Sam would deny he had agreed to anything I wanted and fall back into exactly the same routine as before.

This was not the first time I had suggested we should part, in fact I had often threatened to leave or screamed at Sam to "Get out!" during our frequent rows. I had several times tried to initiate a calm conversation about the subject of amicable separation, but Sam had sabotaged every effort. I began by asking Sam to acknowledge that we could not continue like this, to which he did not reply. I asked him to tell me what he wanted, to which he responded unhelpfully, "I'm just trying to survive." I persevered by suggesting that we should put the house on the market and split the proceeds. Sam's flat "I'm not agreeing to that" did not discourage me. I continued to push and manoeuvre, finally suggesting that I should call an estate agent on Monday, just to find out what the house was worth, and we could take things from there. Sam responded, "Do what you like," which I took to mean that I had his agreement.

Later that day, Sam went to the golf club. I spent a few hours working. Part way through the afternoon, the phone rang, it was my boss Jim, ringing to ask if I would respond to an urgent enquiry from the local radio station the next morning.

Jim and I were deep in conversation when I heard the front door burst open; immediately I became tense and apprehensive. I tried to continue talking to Jim, but I could hear Sam shouting my name in an angry voice and making his way up the stairs towards my office. Sam flung open the door and, provoked rather than stayed by my gesture that I did not want to be disturbed, he flew towards me, thrust his face close to mine and screamed "I've been trying to ring you for a fucking hour!" My whole body was by now crouched in a defensive pose; at the same time I was acutely aware of the desperately embarrassing situation and struggling to retrieve some kind of dignity with Jim, who must have heard everything. Jim made his excuses and ended the call.

My anger and shame were overwhelming. I threw myself at Sam, screaming "How dare you? How fucking dare you?" Sam retaliated by picking up the phone, ripping it from its socket and throwing it across the room. I flew downstairs, grabbed my car keys and ran out of the house. I managed to get away without intervention from Sam, not knowing where I was going, just that I needed to be anywhere but home. There was only one place to go, back to the beach, the crying place. The sanctuary and protection of my car together with the peace of the environment brought the sense of anonymity I craved. I replayed the incident in my mind; what was I going to do? It was unthinkable that I should go back home and try to live some kind of life with Sam after this, and what about my job? I felt so humiliated, how could I have any credibility in my job or the outside world when my life was such a mess?

For a long time, I sat in my car, watching the fading light, yet again completely alone. A vision came, this time a picture of a middle-aged woman staring through the rain-streaked window of a bus, tears falling down her face. Willy Russell's Shirley Valentine, reflecting on the happy times of her early relationship and finally struggling down the bus steps on to the pavement, laden with shopping and proclaiming "I can't remember the day, the week, the month that it happened, when I stopped being....."

I had long remembered that scene, its poignancy and power encapsulating how I felt with unbelievable accuracy. I had nowhere to go, all my things were at home, my clothes and toiletries, my briefcase and the work I needed for tomorrow. Defeated and broken, I drove back to my house and to Sam who just ignored me.

The next day, on arrival at work, Julia told me that Jim had left a message to say he was going to respond to the media and I didn't have to do anything. Once again, I felt a sense of failure and humiliation, all the more acute because I would have to speak to Jim at some point and try to apologise.

Julia made tea and asked me what was wrong. By now relieved to be able to share all my traumas with Julia, I described the scene of the previous day. Julia asked, "what are you going to do?" This was an important question for me; in truth, when such incidents had occurred before, I had done very little, thrown myself into work or a pet project and tried to carry on. I knew that Julia was different, that what she had said on our evening outing about not being prepared to stay where she was threatened or at risk, was true. Julia would have been long gone. What made us so different? Two intelligent, capable women, both able to reason and think logically about the world, yet when faced with challenges in personal relationships, our reactions were poles apart. I wanted so much to be free of this terrible situation, knew I should take decisive action, realised that events were conspiring to bring the whole thing out in the open. In addition to having to deal with the daily trauma of life with Sam, I now also risked my job and my credibility if I didn't do something to change things. Somehow, though, I couldn't see the simple way out.

Julia asked me what I wanted. My reply was instant, "I want to be free, I want to be safe, I want to enjoy my life again and be able to respect myself, without feeling that I'm living a lie and a charade. I want to enjoy the little things that make life worthwhile. I don't see why that's so much to ask; occasional evenings out, a walk on the beach with my partner, mundane and ordinary things like food shopping together and doing the garden."

If only I had realised that all I had to do was believe in myself and all those things would flood back into my life.

14.

CONFESSIONS

*"...the instant you turn that boat toward shore,
you're heading in the direction you want."*

Russ Harris, 'The Happiness Trap'

The next day, I met with Jim. I was dreading the meeting, knowing that I would have to confess more secrets and still very guilty about letting him down over the media contact. We met in Jim's office, he made me a cup of tea, and because he had no idea how to start the conversation, there was an initial awkward silence. To my horror, I began to weep. Jim simply said, "It's OK, I just need to know what you want. It's been obvious to me for some time that things were badly wrong for you at home. You've been distracted and harassed, late for meetings and flustered. All the same, your work is brilliant, and we owe you something, and besides, I consider myself a friend as well as a colleague. We're all human and there are times when we need to ask for help." I was overwhelmed, I hadn't been expecting this.

I didn't really know what to ask for. I told Jim a bit about my problems with Sam, an abridged and heavily edited version, but enough to convey my unhappiness. I said that I wanted to end the relationship and asked Jim if I could come back later with a concrete suggestion, maybe a little time off or at least some part time working hours while I sorted things out. Jim suggested I speak to a staff counsellor and reminded me that the agency had a 'policy' which covered such things.

I felt small and exposed. Many times I had given advice to staff about such matters, believing that it was my place to be strong. My role was to support and advise other people, not to seek such things for myself. Although I was very grateful to Jim, the conversation left me drained and I returned to my office in a haze of misery and humiliation.

A couple of days later, an estate agent came to value the house. I made sure he would be calling when Sam was out, to avoid embarrassment and misunderstanding. He was complimentary about the house, and I was pleasantly surprised at the amount of equity in the property. Sam and I would be able to split the proceeds of the sale and still live comfortably.

Later that evening, I took a deep breath and raised the subject of the valuation with Sam, hoping for a sensible conversation about what we should do next. Immediately Sam was furious and dismissive, he denied having agreed to any such thing and refused to discuss the matter further. I tried to remind him of our conversation about selling the house, but he was unshakeable. My plans once again in disarray, I thought I was going mad. So many conversations with Sam ended this way, either he denied having agreed to the things I wanted or he simply refused to engage in reasoned debate. Once again defeated and frustrated, I went to bed early with my book.

The next day, my mobile phone rang. It was a number I didn't recognise. I answered to find that it was Liz, "I thought you were going to ring me." I was momentarily taken aback and stumbled over my words, feeling irrationally that I had done something wrong. Eventually I regained my composure and apologised to Liz, citing the demands of work and consequent exhaustion as my reasons for failing to call as promised.

Liz wanted to know what had been happening, what progress I had made. Feeling a little defensive, I explained about my conversations with Sam, the estate agent and my meeting with Jim. I could not bear to recount the incident when Sam had screamed at me during my phone call to Jim, so left that out. Liz, with characteristic insight, pointed out that I had done lots of things, but I was still there. She encouraged me to do something more decisive and reminded me that the situation was far from safe and I could well get badly hurt. Liz encouraged me to simply get out, pack a suitcase, get into the car and go somewhere safe. Given the support I had from work and Jim's offer of help I could hardly be in a better position to take action.

After the phone call I sat in silence for a while. I knew that Liz was right, everything was conspiring to support me in taking decisive action. My cover had been broken despite my attempts to hide everything from the outside world, and the response had been nothing but supportive. Yet there was a hesitation I couldn't explain. Above all I wanted to be free and safe, but the reticence, which in retrospect I can only summarise as a combination of fear and habit, held me back.

For the next few weeks, I played and replayed the conversation with Liz in my mind, but instead of taking her advice and simply leaving I decided I wanted to sort out practical matters first. I applied to the bank and discovered that I could obtain sufficient mortgage in my own right to buy Sam out of the house. I didn't want to leave my home and my possessions and face a protracted wrangle over money.

With characteristic false optimism, I somehow imagined that Sam would simply agree to and comply with my plan. Would I never learn?

15.

STEVE AGAIN

"Truth be told I've tried my best,
But somewhere along the way,
I got caught up in all there was to offer
And the cost was so much more than I could bear"

Sarah Mclachlan, 'Fallen'

Steve and I were due to meet the day before my course. The venue was far enough from home to justify an overnight stay, I had arranged an extra night at the hotel and Steve had booked into a nearby B&B. We agreed to meet at lunchtime on the day before the course.

We met for lunch in a country pub, taking a walk around the pretty village afterwards. We found ourselves trying to unravel the tangle which had resulted in our eventual loss of contact. Wanting to delay the inevitable discussion about me and Sam, I asked Steve about his relationship with Faye. The Steve I used to know so well would compartmentalise impeccably, keeping his relationship with Faye so private that I had imagined it to be a stable and loving partnership which he sought to protect at all costs, in contrast to his friendship with me, which I assumed Steve regarded as a 'bit of fun'. In consequence, I had always believed that no matter what I might have meant to Steve, I would always be second to Faye in his affections, a concept which had allowed me to distance myself emotionally from him yet enjoy his company.

I was surprised, therefore, with Steve's openness. He explained that, for a while before her death, he and Faye had grown apart. He expressed regret that their relationship ended before she really understood that he loved her. I was deeply moved by Steve's revelations. Never before had I heard him talk of love, except in jest.

If I was taken aback at Steve's revelations about his relationship with Faye, I was astounded when he said, "And my regret about the way you and I lost contact is that I don't think you ever understood that I also loved you." I was quite literally lost for words. At the same time, I knew immediately what Steve meant. This was no declaration of undying romantic love, no cheap attempt to seduce me, but a genuine and pure expression of love from one person to another. I also knew instantly that I had loved him too. Ironically, the openness of our friendship and the absence of the frantic and temporary sense of all embracing, gut wrenching obsession which so often characterises the beginning of romantic liaisons had allowed me to see him as a whole person, for good and ill. For once, in a relationship with a man, my life pattern hadn't taken over. I knew his foibles and irritations as well as I knew his endearing and captivating qualities, but never stopped to recognise that I loved him because of, not despite these things.

When Sam came along, sweeping me up into a disorientating fog of charm and charisma, there had been no contest. Even if Steve had openly declared himself a serious rival to Sam for my affections, I would, at that moment, have chosen Sam.

I asked Steve why he didn't tell me all this before, I had thought I didn't matter to him. He said that I could be forgiven for that and took his share of the responsibility for losing touch. After Faye's death he had been overwhelmed with grief and spent a great deal of time working through his feelings. We both acknowledged that, had we tried to start a relationship at that time, it would have been doomed.

I had thought I knew Steve well, thought that he was flippant and child-like, not capable of deep emotion. Now I realised how wrong I had been; Steve felt things very deeply, he simply didn't express them very well. With a sense of bitter irony, I realised that I had mistaken Sam's grandiose and superficial displays of affection and attention for genuine love, whilst ignoring and rejecting Steve's persistence and loyalty.

I knew that Steve's candour deserved my reciprocation. I responded to his "So what about you? Why did you stop returning my calls?" with as honest a response as I could summon. "When I met Sam, I was afraid of being lonely. I hadn't lived alone before and I never gave myself a chance to find out if I could cope. He was charming and gregarious and I guess I thought I had met the love of my life. I was sick of deceit, I was never proud of my affair with you and when I found out that Joe had also been cheating on me, everything felt sordid. At that time, it just seemed important to me to find a partnership that was untainted, someone to whom I could be faithful and loyal, without the baggage." As I spoke the words, they sounded hollow, like a story which had never held credence, even when I thought I believed it.

Steve asked what went wrong and I said that Sam could see no good in me. Steve was incredulous. With a sense of weariness, I encapsulated quickly as much of my story as I could bear to tell again. Every time I went back over this stuff, it drained me more. I began to cry a little; Steve pulled me towards him and said gently "No matter what happens between us, you have to get out of this."

16.

WEEKEND AGAIN

"I have sunk so low, I messed up,
Better I should know..."

Sarah Mclachlan, 'Fallen'

Although I had sometimes shared my frustrations with Sam's daughter, Helen, I had felt justified in doing so because she was already aware of her father's behaviour and I was in dire need of the support of someone who understood what I was going through. I had never, however, confided in my family, trying desperately to keep up a facade and petrified of humiliation.

My brother and his wife occasionally came to stay, though their visits had become less frequent. At first my brother had liked Sam very much. They established some social contact and even spent occasional golf weekends together. Although Sam instantly reverted to his old self, gregarious and chatty, with his friends and family, during visits from my family his behaviour had begun to deteriorate and cracks had begun to show. I was therefore apprehensive when my brother and his wife came for the weekend.

Sam was less than enthusiastic about the visit and refused to discuss plans for an outing. I organised meals and made the house cosy and comfortable without his help. When our visitors arrived, Sam was a little off-hand and I found myself uneasy and couldn't relax. The first evening was lack lustre but passed without incident. The following day I suggested that we go to the beach, but again Sam was unenthusiastic. The outing was uninspiring and I could tell that everyone sensed an atmosphere.

When we returned, I began to plan the evening meal. I offered everyone a glass of wine; Sam refused, intending to drink wine with dinner. The meal almost ready, just before asking everyone to the table I refilled glasses, also taking Sam a glass as we were about to eat. Without warning he exploded, screaming that he had said he didn't want wine until dinner and asking my brother for confirmation. I was devastated; the shock of such exposure after years of pretending left me shaking and humiliated. I tried, pathetically, to serve dinner without showing a reaction. Inevitably I only made matters worse. I began to sob uncontrollably, acutely aware of our guests' embarrassment. Just as he had done in the presence of his daughter, Sam ignored me completely and carried on talking as though nothing had happened. It was as though I was some slave to be chastised for a misdemeanour then dismissed. Of all the incidents I had experienced, this was the most humiliating; I had never felt so demeaned and embarrassed.

Somehow, we got through the evening and my relatives left the next day. As we parted, my brother whispered, "Ring me."

Believing that even Sam would not let an incident such as this pass without making amends, I expected him to ring my brother and apologise. I even suggested this to him; he flatly refused. Somehow, I had still been hoping that the situation could be retrieved and the false security of my secrecy restored. Following Sam's refusal, I rang my brother. For the first time, we had an honest conversation. I confessed everything, seeing no other way to proceed. My brother was very candid, he said that they had become increasingly concerned about Sam's behaviour and they had noticed that I had become withdrawn and my personality suppressed. They had continued to visit out of duty, thinking that I would have said something if I needed help. At the end of the conversation, my brother said he had heard enough, and suggested I leave immediately.

17.

ESCAPE

"This is really not my home."

Cara Dillon, 'Garden Valley'

For weeks after my brother's visit I was tortured with the desperation to leave. My brother rang frequently on my mobile phone at prearranged times, with words of encouragement which Sam could not interrupt, yet I still did not have the courage to go.

One day I came home from work to find Sam, head in hands, crying like a small child, still in his dressing gown. At first, he refused to speak to me, when I persisted he complained of pains in his chest. I was familiar with this scenario, Sam was convinced that he had or was going to develop heart problems. He had been through many tests and investigations, all negative, none of which reassured him. He was convinced that next time it would be the real thing.

The conversation took on a familiar format. I asked Sam to describe his symptoms, I tried to sympathise then suggested that he should go and see the doctor. Sam became distressed and enraged, refusing to consult the GP and blaming me for being unhelpful. I did not believe that Sam was seriously ill. I knew that anyone with chest pains should consult a doctor, the most obvious course of action. I also knew that Sam had a history of panic attacks, that the thought of becoming ill frightened him and that he couldn't work out what to do. As a result, he became anxious and aggressive, sharing his anxieties only with me and occasionally with the doctor, resulting in the periodic battery of tests to which he was subjected. Whichever way I played things, the scenario always ended the same. Sam inexplicably blamed me for his woes; I became angry and told him to get some help because nothing I said or did seemed to satisfy him. I felt alone and exasperated.

Sam went back to bed protesting that he couldn't eat. An hour later I took him some dinner, all of which he consumed. The next day was Sam's golf club day. He got up early and went out as usual, without mention of the previous day's trauma.

Over the past few months I had begun to feel ill. I was constantly exhausted, my body ached, some days I could hardly struggle out of bed, my limbs didn't seem to want to work. I suffered from headaches, frequently caught colds and other bugs and recent tests had shown I had an auto-immune system deficiency. Sam was unsympathetic, believing that I did not deserve his support because I had no understanding for his needs. I knew that the stress of my life-style was a major cause of my symptoms, that if I didn't do something to change things I risked more serious illness.

Several times I had broached the subject of separation, suggesting I could buy Sam out of the house. At times there were signs of recognition in Sam that we could not continue as we were, but the old pattern replayed again and again and he either denied having agreed to anything or refused to make the next move.

I recognised that my persistent efforts to reason with Sam were never likely to bring about the results I wanted. Despite Sam's obvious unhappiness, he just wanted our lives to carry on as they always had. After all, his practical needs were catered for, his bills were paid and he had established for himself a comfortable and enjoyable social life at the golf club. I also knew that something about our unhealthy power relationship fed Sam's distorted need for dominance and possession.

At the suggestion of Liz, I rang my close friend Lucy. I had never confessed my unhappiness to Lucy, despite the longevity of our friendship. Lucy had been married for many years to Peter, their close and easy relationship constantly reminding me of the inadequacies of my own. Feeling inferior and embarrassed, I had feigned normality and hidden my distress. I asked her to meet me, knowing that she would sense my need and not hesitate.

Once again, I found myself describing the desperate situation with Sam. Lucy was horrified, clearly feared for my safety and, as I knew she would, offered to do anything she could to help. This time I swallowed my pride and asked if I could use Lucy's house as my retreat. I would also be closer to my family, able to tell them in person what was happening and visit them at Christmas. We agreed that I would arrange to take some time away from work, then simply pack my case and slip away.

It was three weeks before Christmas. I had spoken to Jim and it was agreed that from the end of the following week I would take leave, meaning I could return to work in the New Year. Julia had asked me to come and stay with her when I returned, while our property was sorted out. I was apprehensive about leaving my home, this wasn't what I wanted. I was by no means clear how I was going to get Sam to cooperate in the sale of the house and sharing of its proceeds. Nevertheless, the thought of breaking away from this terrible pattern and becoming free from Sam's tyranny was compelling, so I stuck to the plan.

Steve had now begun to ring weekly. He was his normal, chatty, affable self. A few days before I was due to make my escape, he rang me at work. Faced with a million tasks to organise before I took my leave I felt pressurised and out of control. Steve was trying to arrange another meeting between us, but his cheerful "Are you coming out to play?" struck the wrong note. I flew back at him: "Can't you ever be serious? This is the most difficult thing I have ever had to do and all you are interested in is messing around." Steve understood the situation but was obviously a little hurt; he suggested that some time away might help me get through this. I was even more incredulous at Steve's naivety, how could he imagine that I would be free so easily? This was only the beginning. I put him off, promising to arrange something after Christmas but feeling that I just couldn't deal with Steve at the moment, he was complicating things and his attempts to arrange a meeting were a pressure I could do without.

The night before I was due to make my getaway I packed my case and hid it in the boot of my car. I woke early the next morning, made tea as usual then told Sam I needed to call at the shop for something I had forgotten. I didn't stop to wait for his response. I was out of the front door and in my car as quickly as I could manage. My hands were sweaty and trembling and I had trouble getting the key into the ignition. Finally, the engine started and my car began to move. I didn't dare look back in case Sam was coming after me, knowing that this was just an irrational fear; he would probably still be reading the paper in bed.

I drove for fifty miles before I allowed myself to stop for a much needed cup of coffee. I rang Sam. I didn't know what to expect when he picked up the phone, whether he would be angry or anxious that I had not returned, but he was matter of fact, even disinterested in where I was. His mood swings and inconsistency never failed to leave me confused and disorientated and fuelled my many fears. I told him I was leaving; there was no reply for a few seconds, then he said, "Ok I'll wait to hear from you." That was it! How could he change from a controlling dictator who monitored my every move to a cold and disinterested bystander?

It was a strange journey. Still haunted by the vestiges of fear which accompanied my departure from home, I was also experiencing a perplexing sense of confusion, I had wanted to feel free and exhilarated but the sensation just wouldn't come. I realised that, on a superficial level at least, my feelings had become habitual; I had been trapped in the cycle of fear, apprehension, disappointment and frustration for so long it was going to take a while to work through this.

I stopped off a couple of times on my journey, revelling in the freedom and enjoying my own company. I needed the protracted journey to begin to settle my thoughts and allow some time for the fear to subside.

18.

GOOD FRIENDS

*"Beauty I'd always missed with these eyes before,
Just what the truth is I can't say any more"*

The Moody Blues, 'Nights in White Satin'

I had known Lucy for more than twenty years. Until I met Sam, we saw each other frequently and spoke almost daily on the phone. Lucy is a powerful and confident person. She and Peter have been married since their late teens and their relationship is solid. Despite the closeness of our friendship, I had been reticent to confide too much in Lucy over the years about my traumas and problems. I had always somehow felt inferior to Lucy; in the face of my friend's perceived security and stability, I had tried to present an outward impression that all was well.

When I met Sam, I had been desperate for Lucy to approve of him. At first, we had shared some social contact with Lucy and Peter. Wanting to create a good impression, Sam had been outwardly charming and affable. Gradually, though, Sam became critical of Lucy and Peter, ultimately refusing to meet up with them. I made excuses and my contact with Lucy gradually diminished to the occasional phone call when Sam was not there. Our move to the south had provided welcome relief from the strain of having to cover up. During the past three years, Lucy and I had spoken only a couple of times.

I arrived at Lucy and Peter's house in the darkening afternoon. The rooms were softly lit and welcoming, the picture of a long and comfortable habitation. Lucy and Peter seemed to coexist so effortlessly, their gentle banter never stopping. Peter was kind and laid-back, accepting my presence in his home as naturally as Lucy's. We had become very easy and relaxed together over the years; it took only an instant for that familiar sense of safety and protection, absent for so long, to return.

The evening was everything I needed. We drank a little wine, ate some good food, played some music and talked. Lucy's capacity to listen and support me seemed endless. When I finally went to bed, despite my exhaustion I couldn't sleep. It was almost overwhelming to be in such a safe and convivial place after the harshness of the past few years. With a sense of poignancy and sadness, I lay in the darkness involuntarily replaying scenes from my relationships, realising that I had never felt the sense of easy security and compatibility enjoyed by Lucy and Peter, I wondered if I ever would. I finally fell asleep in the early hours, haunted by the familiar dream of travelling on a bus driven by my father. This time no one on the bus was laughing at me, the visionary journey passed in peace as I watched the beautiful countryside through the window.

The next morning, I was brought tea in bed, told to take as long as I liked to get myself up and ready and enjoy a long hot bath if I wanted to. Such kindness, yet only what everyone deserved. I knew that, given my freedom, I could do the same; make my friends and relations welcome in my home, relax and enjoy their company, cook food for them and allow myself to experience the variety and spontaneity which had been missing for so long.

I spent the next few days catching up on sleep, wandering around shops, talking to Lucy and generally allowing myself at last to relax and feel safe. I then went to visit my brother and his wife who were very supportive, having seen Sam's behaviour first hand.

Gradually I began to feel a little more secure, more in control of my life. Even in Sam's absence though, the fear still persisted. I was aware of a subtle undercurrent of anxiety, a feeling that I should be somewhere else, meet some deadline or complete some task in order to avoid Sam's wrath. I realised that my pattern would be difficult to break, its coded message ran like DNA through my system, deep and entrenched. The urge to manage my environment, to take on responsibility for the behaviour of others in a desperate struggle to regain a sense of peace and security long since absent from my life, was invasive and all-consuming. I knew that Liz was right, only Sam was responsible for his behaviour. I could not change him and he could not love me; but this was not about Sam. I knew that I had to do more than simply walk away, that the pattern could repeat at any time. I had somehow to find a way to believe that I was worth more than this struggle, to reach inside to the desperate wounded child who had never recovered from the loss of her father's support and affection and help her to heal.

19.

SAM AGAIN

"Fools, they thought I was all right,
They couldn't see that I was dying inside"

Judy Truce, 'Ladies' Night'

It took ten days for Sam to ring. I saw my home number on the screen of my mobile phone and decided I should answer; we would have to communicate eventually. Sam was crying, making dramatic faltering sounds and pausing for long periods between sobs. He wanted to know why I had just left in that way, without explanation, and whether I was coming back for Christmas, now only two days away. I felt unemotional and detached. I reminded Sam that I had tried to reason and negotiate with him without success and I had to make a decision about what to do for myself, or nothing would change. He told me he was lonely and insisted that I should come back home for Christmas, he would buy the food, even cook for me. I was firm and consistent. I would not be coming home, we would have to talk in the New Year, sort out the practicalities. He asked if he could ring on Christmas day to which I agreed, wanting to end the conversation.

I went shopping alone. I had known that Sam would ring but had no idea what he would say. What had taken him so long? What had he been doing for ten days? As I wandered around the smart and attractive town with its small alleyways and cobbled streets, I began to think of Steve. I had been unkind to him last time we spoke, yet I knew I hadn't deterred my friend, he was simply allowing me some space to work things out. I owed him a phone call. I made my way to the river. The weather was beautiful, crisp, cold and sunlit. I sat on a bench and rang Steve's number, hoping to catch him in. Relieved and delighted to hear Steve's voice, I apologised for my rudeness during our previous conversation. Steve was good humoured and understanding "I can be a bit thoughtless sometimes, I deserved your irritation. Anyway, more importantly, how are you?" We talked for nearly an hour. It was so easy to talk to Steve, to make him laugh and to laugh with him. Of course, he wanted to arrange a meeting. He suggested that, once I was settled in Julia's house, we should meet for a weekend break in the country. I accepted his offer and Steve promised to do some digging around for the right place. He was off to spend Christmas with his sister on the south coast and we agreed to talk between Christmas and New Year.

I went back to town. After a coffee and sandwich, I browsed a little more. In a small card shop down a winding alley, I discovered a beautiful card with a local scene showing part of the river near where I had sat talking to Steve. I realised that I had forgotten to send Steve a Christmas card and bought it for him, mentally composing the note I would enclose, thanking him for his patience and friendship.

I went out to visit my family, distributing presents on Christmas Eve, spending Christmas Day with my son and his partner. It had been very difficult to tell my son what had been happening between Sam and me. I had so wanted him to feel that I had settled down and found a stable relationship after separating from his father. His initial approval of Sam was one of the things which persuaded me that it was a good idea to stay with Sam. My son had never lived with us, so his impression was that Sam was affable and charming, a façade Sam had continued to present directly to my son, but in his absence Sam became critical and dismissive of him and jealous of our relationship. In consequence, having to confess to the truth was extremely difficult; I felt as though he might not believe me and somehow as though I had failed him as a mother and a role model.

He was, however, understanding and reassuring, even offering to speak to Sam himself, an offer I politely declined.

After lunch on Christmas Day my phone rang, it was Sam. I went into the garden to take the call. Sam was more composed, making an attempt to be charming and affectionate. He was spending Christmas Day with his daughter, Helen. I asked what Sam had told Helen and how she had reacted to the news of my departure. Sam gave some vague response and I suspected he had made some excuse, failed to tell Helen what was actually happening. Sam sounded a little more like the man I had first met. He was apologetic, told me how much he missed me and how he wished we were spending Christmas together, just the two of us. Sam said he knew he had treated me very badly and pleaded with me to give him another chance. Despite myself, I found I was crying. It had been a long time since I had heard any gentleness or genuine feeling in Sam's voice. He sounded just like the man I had fallen in love with. I told him to try and enjoy the holiday and promised to ring in a few days' time.

On Boxing Day, I was invited to my niece, Emily's house. Emily is a charming and gregarious young woman. She and her partner have two small children. Emily greeted me at the door, quickly thrusting a glass of mulled wine at me and leading me into a colourful kitchen filled with food and the noise of excited children.

Josh and Emily are great parents, I got the impression that they set out to make the lives of their children a joy every day. I was touched by their patience and inventiveness, the way they diverted fractious and overwrought children into calmer pursuits, organised simple and stimulating games and activities which adults and children could enjoy together and still seemed relaxed and easy with each other.

Although the day was cold it was sunny and dry and Emily had been determined to make the most of the outside space. The French windows were open onto a small patio which contained a lit chimenea and barbecue. The low wall bordering the patio was laid out with tea lights in coloured glass jars and the area was decorated with silver frosting and tinsel, finished with home-made decorations. The scene was almost unbelievably harmonious, like a stylised picture of Christmas portrayed in the most evocative advertisements or sentimental films. Suddenly I found the whole experience overwhelming; I was struck by the most poignant and devastating sense of loss and sadness. *I* had a lovely house, *I* knew how to make people welcome, *I* could do all this! Like the time I had sat by the beach, watching the family playing together and imagining I was in a goldfish bowl, I experienced a sense of detachment and unreality. It was as though I was denied the opportunity to take part in a blissful existence enjoyed by all those around me, condemned by some past misdemeanour to watch but never to experience the joy for myself. Realising I was about to burst into tears and desperate to avoid embarrassment, I walked quickly outside and sat on the low wall, my back to the French windows, staring at the garden. I managed to choke back the tears but did not dare return to the lounge. I stayed there for a long time, watching the candles and trying to relax. Suddenly someone was beside me. I turned to see Emily's gently smiling face, "Can I join you?" I nodded, sensing that Emily knew intuitively what I was going through.

She asked if I wanted to talk. I explained that I didn't want to spoil the party, I just wanted to get away for a while, I guess the whole thing had just got to me. Emily said nothing, sitting very still and close.

I realised that I needed very much to tell someone how I was feeling. Despite the kindness of my friends and close relatives I had not wanted to burden them with my problems. Although I liked Emily very much, our relationship was not close and somehow I felt safe expressing my thoughts to her. As I talked I realised just how confused I was, how torn I felt and how burdened I was by the choices I needed to make.

I found myself spilling out the whole story. I told her that that things between me and Sam had become intolerable and I had to do something to break away. I explained how I hid myself away because I was ashamed of another failure, I wanted to keep up the pretence that Sam and I had a happy life. I explained that it was hard to walk away from the things I had worked for, the familiar surroundings, books and music. I told her I was intending to move in temporarily with my friend Julia but I didn't know whether I would get access to my things and there wasn't room for much in Julia's tiny house. I said I was worried about paying the bills and covering the mortgage so the house wouldn't be repossessed and I didn't think Sam would pay for anything. I told her that running away like this had only postponed what I had to do. I said I still had to reason with Sam, try to get things moving so I could have some independence and start to live my life again and I didn't know how long that would take. I told her I'd always been envious of the happy and peaceful existence she and Josh had and didn't believe that would ever happen to me. I stopped; Emily touched my arm and sat with me a while longer. She didn't speak, didn't comment on my somewhat idealised impression of her life. Emily didn't need to say anything, I guess she knew she was lucky, some people just were.

The conversation unnerved me; suddenly I wasn't sure I'd made the right decision by running away and leaving everything I'd worked for all my life. I began to question whether leaving Sam was the right thing to do. I was glad to get back to Lucy and Peter's house. I explained that I was very tired and went to bed straight away.

20.

SECOND THOUGHTS

*"What looked like morning was the
beginning of endless night."*

William Peter Blatty, 'The Exorcist'

The next morning, I woke very early. My mind was spinning, I wondered how I could have allowed myself to retreat like this; I had responsibilities, a house and a job. What had I done to Sam? We had been together a long time, he deserved better than this. He had sounded so sorry and so lonely on Christmas Day, surely my actions must have had a profound impact on him and made him see that we needed to sort out our relationship to try to find some happiness together. He really sounded as though he had finally developed some insight, that the shock of my departure had made him realise that he needed to change his behaviour. I didn't want to live with Julia, I had my own lovely home, a place I had worked for. I was sure I could reason with Sam, get him to book a holiday, spend some money on the house and take me out occasionally. I had to go home straight away and sort this out.

When Lucy put her head around my bedroom door she found me dressed and packed, ready to go. Lucy was shocked and instantly concerned, she asked what I was doing. I was distracted and anxious; I knew I had to face Lucy and explain and had been dreading this moment. "I have to go home, Lucy. I can't just let things drift like this. There is money and property to sort out and I have to speak to Sam face to face." I did not confess my thoughts about wanting to put things right with Sam; I knew Lucy would try to dissuade me. Lucy urged me to come and sit down, have some tea and we could talk this over. I didn't want to do this but agreed because I knew Lucy was anxious. We talked for a while. Lucy told me that whatever happened she would be there for me, advised me that she didn't think it was a good idea for me to go home, but respected my decision. She made me promise to ring daily, knowing how easy it would be for me to become lost and trapped again in a fraught and dangerous situation. But I just did not seem to see the danger; I was adamant that I would be OK and convinced I could talk to Sam and find some resolution.

I rang my brother to tell him about my decision to return home, carefully omitting my second thoughts about Sam. Even so, he was horrified, convinced that Sam would try to persuade me to stay. He tried hard to dissuade me, but I asked him to trust me and promised to keep in touch.

I left my son a brief voicemail, relieved that I didn't have to speak directly to him.

I drove down the motorway too fast, anxious to get back as soon as possible. I stopped a couple of times, trying to ring Sam, who still didn't know I was coming back, but there was no answer. I imagined Sam greeting me with relief and overjoyed to see me. I pictured us talking about our lives, eating the meal Sam had promised to cook for me, walking on the beach together. I remembered the card I had bought for Steve but still not sent, and decided I would give it to Sam, it was the least I could do after I had ruined his Christmas.

21.

HOMECOMING

"Noble silence gives us the chance to recognise how our habit energy manifests in the ways we react to people and situations around us ...we are able to transform our ways of responding to any number of situations. This silence is called noble because it has the power to heal. When you practise noble silence you aren't just refraining from talking; you're calming and quietening your thinking. You're turning off radio non-stop thinking."

Thich Nhat Hanh, 'Silence'

When I arrived home, Sam was still not there. I couldn't think where he could be. I had imagined him distraught and helpless, spending most of his time in bed and not bothering to get dressed or go out. The house was cold, but tidy and neat. There was food in the fridge and the remains of a fire in the grate.

I made myself a drink and sat in the conservatory, waiting. Eventually, Sam's car drew up the drive. I watched him from the window; he had obviously been to the golf club and was unloading his equipment and returning it to the garage. He had clearly seen my car but was making no move to hurry inside and greet me.

Eventually he opened the front door. He glanced in my direction and said, "When did you get here?" There was no smile, no attempt to touch me and my overall impression was that he was indifferent to my presence.

Sam went around the house doing routine tasks, taking his time, while I waited patiently for him to come and talk to me. When he made no move to join me, I offered to make coffee and asked him to come and talk. It was clear that, without my intervention, Sam would have carried on where we had left off, emotionally detached and disinterested. I could not believe that after all he had said to me on the phone on Christmas Day, this was his reaction to my return.

We sat together in silence at first; I didn't know how to begin the conversation and I felt the return of the familiar feeling of apprehension, knowing that I must choose my words very carefully so as not to provoke the wrong reaction from Sam. In time we began to communicate. Sam wanted to know why I had chosen to leave in the way that I did. I explained that I had tried so hard to get him to discuss our relationship, without success, and I could think of no other way to make him realise that something needed to be done. I asked what he had been doing while I was away. Sam did not ask about where I had been or who I had seen.

We began to drift into familiar deep water. I started to detail all the things I felt were wrong with our relationship and all the things I wanted us to do to put it right. Sam responded by complaining that I never showed him sympathy and understanding. I asked him what he wanted; did he want the relationship to work? He simply said, "It takes two." We were getting nowhere, nothing about this discussion felt different, my departure seemed incidental, it might never have happened. Still I could not let go, knowing that Sam would have happily stopped talking, turned on the TV and waited for me to make a meal, I grasped at the captive audience I now had with Sam and carried on talking, trying every angle I could think of to get him to make constructive suggestions. I moved on to practical issues. What about the jobs which needed doing around the house? What about booking a holiday? Could we at least go out for dinner and discuss things over a relaxed meal? Sam was non-committal about my requests and flatly refused to go out for dinner.

Finally, after a make-shift meal prepared by me, eaten in silence, I went to bed. Exhausted after the long drive and once again frustrated by Sam's unpredictable and obstructive behaviour, I fell asleep quickly, waking at first light to find Sam beside me in bed.

The next day I tried again to engage Sam in a constructive dialogue. I had by now lost all perspective. Instead of asking myself what I really wanted then taking action, I gave all the decision-making power over to Sam. I asked him repeatedly to say whether he wanted the relationship to continue. How could we improve things? If we were to separate, what was the most constructive and least painful way of making this happen? Sam was vague and uncooperative. In the end, we began to bicker, then to have a full-scale row. The usual stuff came up, Sam's ability to change his behaviour dramatically when he was with people he wanted to impress, my 'betrayal' when Helen and Tom last visited, Sam's lack of willingness to contribute financially or practically to the running of the household and my extravagance. It went on and on. Ultimately, we degenerated into a strained silence, which lasted for the next couple of days.

There were messages on my phone from my brother, my son, Lucy and Steve, none of whom I had contacted since returning home. I knew I should ring them but didn't have the heart. I was becoming depressed and sinking deeper into the well, couldn't face explanations and feeling that I had let everyone down. There was also a message from Julia, still expecting me to be coming to stay in the New Year. What was I going to do?

The next day, I decided to make one more attempt to get Sam to talk, what had I got to lose? Once again, I tried to find out what he wanted to do, did he want us to separate? If so, how were we going to deal with the practicalities? Was there an alternative, could we put things right? Sam began to hint that he didn't want us to separate. I seized on this, a breakthrough at last. I started to talk about how I wanted our relationship to work. Could we plan outings? Spend money on the house? Go away together? This time Sam seemed willing to concede a little.

We began to talk about money. For many years, we had operated separate accounts. I rarely discussed money with Sam, except to try and get him to agree to spend some of our savings on home improvements, which he persistently refused to do. In an effort to keep the peace and appease Sam by providing all the things he wanted, I had often overstretched myself financially. I had run up a large credit card debt which Sam didn't know about and which preyed on my mind. Sam now seemed to be amenable to my suggestion of home improvements and I asked him how much he was willing to spend. He mentioned a modest amount and I fetched a pen and paper, eager for a constructive dialogue at last. I decided that I better come clean and confess to my credit card debt, in the hope that Sam would agree to pay it off from our savings.

Without warning, Sam exploded; his anger was so intense that I physically recoiled at its suddenness and ferocity. He accused me of being deceitful, demanded to know if I had a secret lover on whom I had lavished money or if I had spent it on my son. He called me a whore and a liar. I flew back at him, screaming that he had taken me for granted, sponged off me, expected me to pay for everything while he contributed nothing, never treated me or took me out, spent all his money on his car and the golf club, neither of which I was invited to share with him. The recriminations went on and on. I knew that if I pushed Sam too far I would be in physical danger; I stopped just short of what I judged to be the point of no return, grabbed my handbag and keys and flew out of the door.

Two weeks before, I would never have imagined I would be back at the crying beach, but here I sat, once again in the goldfish bowl. I had made an escape, felt safe and relieved, put my plan into action; now it felt like I had never been away. What was I going to do? I was letting so many people down; Lucy, Jim, Julia, my relatives, they had all put themselves out to help me sort things; and what about Steve? I had promised to phone him, agreed that we could have a weekend together in the New Year. I could still contact Julia and move in with her, today if necessary, but what about my own house? If I left Sam there, I was afraid he wouldn't pay the bills and it would be repossessed. If I walked away, how could I ever get Sam to cooperate in sorting out the finances? If I couldn't do that, how could I ever be independent?

Despite the obvious danger and the terrible state of my relationship with Sam, things which should have given me absolute clarity, I simply couldn't see what any sane person should have seen. I didn't know what I wanted, didn't know what to do, felt confused and alone, unable to speak to my friends and utterly helpless. I knew that I would never be able to sort things out with Sam, his mood swings and inconsistency made him impossible to reason with. I couldn't believe how naive I had been, going back to that awful situation, putting myself at risk and believing that Sam could change. I knew that I could have talked to Lucy or Julia, that both of them would have provided the sweet voice of reason, but I wanted to talk to someone who really knew Sam, who knew first-hand what I was going through. In desperation, I decided to ring Helen, remembering our conversation of a few months back and Helen's words of support. Surely Helen would know what to do, perhaps she could reason with her father on my behalf, encourage him to see sense?

Helen was a little breathless, as though under pressure to meet some deadline, her distracted "Hello?" wrong-footed me and I began to stumble over my words, not really sure what I wanted to say. "Helen, I hope you don't mind me ringing, I just need to talk to someone who really understands what's going on between me and your Dad." There was silence on the other end; I continued, "Remember you said you wanted me to let you know what was happening, that you might be able to help?" Helen's reply was distant, a little cold, "I remember our conversation, yes." I felt a sense of wrongness, as though I was bothering Helen, that the conversation was futile and a little embarrassing. I had little option but to continue, finish what I had started. "I wondered, I hoped, I just wanted to do what you said I should, to tell you what's happening and ask for your help. You must know about what happened over Christmas. Well, I went back to try and sort things out with your Dad and it all became difficult again. I wondered whether you could do something, perhaps talk to him?" Helen's reply was curt, "Look, I know what I said and I do sympathise, but I think you have to sort this out yourself. No amount of talking has ever made a difference to my father. I told you I believed you needed to get out and if things are that bad then that's what you must do. I have my own life and my own stress; I just can't cope with him as well." I felt humiliated and let down, hadn't Helen promised to help? I apologised for bothering Helen and finished the conversation.

I had never felt so alone. Unbelievably, even after all I had experienced, even though I had the clear support of my friends and family and the opportunity to improve my life beyond recognition by walking away, I was still hoping for someone to "fix" Sam. Instead of realising that all I had to do was change *my* behaviour, I was still under some delusion that there was someone or something that could change Sam to make me happy.

Still stinging from Helen's rebuke, I felt a sense of unreality, a tingling numbness which invaded my consciousness, enveloping me in a kind of sticky web, like a fly caught by a spider. I felt trapped and helpless. I couldn't go home yet, there was something I needed to reach, something hovering before my vision, foggy and indistinct, like a ghost I was compelled to follow, or maybe just an external representation of my soul. Somehow I knew that it was a symbol of the solution to my terrible confusion, a phantom I had to make real before it could all fall into place.

Almost instinctively, I drove to a nearby small town. It was a place with a spiritual feel, where I could buy unusual books, aromatic oils, health foods and pretty jewellery. I went there sometimes to lose myself in the ambience of peace and gentleness, so absent from my life. I walked up the high street in a daze, not sure where I was going, but luxuriating in the refuge of anonymity. I had once visited a tarot reader here, seeking reassurance I couldn't find in my day to day existence. He had foretold many tears, but said that ultimately, I would be happy. I had interpreted this to mean that Sam and I would eventually put things right. In desperation I decided to consult the tarot reader again but found that he was no longer there. Outside the shop where the reading had taken place was a pile of second hand books in a cardboard box. I picked up a book on meditation, which fell open at a page with only one sentence:

"In silence we can know God"

I began to cry. Why couldn't I see what I needed to do? Couldn't anyone help me? I returned to the car, always my sanctuary and means of escape. I sat in the driver's seat, closed my eyes and finally released the terrible burden I was carrying. I hoped that whatever higher power existed, it would hear my silent prayer, accept my burden and do what needed to be done.

When I returned home, Sam's car was gone. I sat in silence, dreading his return, not knowing what was going to happen next, only that it was out of my hands, I had nothing left inside. A few hours later, Sam came through the door. Instead of ignoring me as usual, he came and sat next to me on the sofa. I heard him take a breath and turned towards him. He began to speak "I've made a decision. I have a friend at the golf club who has a flat in the harbour which he lets out and he's willing for me to stay there at a very low rent. You can do what you like with the house, buy me out or sell. I'll leave it to you. I know you will be honourable about the money." I was stunned, never before had Sam taken the initiative in our relationship; I had no idea what had prompted him to change, but the sense of relief was overwhelming. I hardly dared to speak, in case I might break the spell. I knew without doubt that this was what I wanted. I simply hadn't been able to break away and make the decision myself.

Incredibly, after all my efforts, arguments with myself and agonising, it was Sam, cruel, inconsistent, indifferent Sam, who had made the final decision that we should part. It seemed that the Universe had answered my prayer in the most perplexing way.

I began to weep; Sam put his hand on my shoulder, we pulled together and cried in each other's arms. Finally, we could talk reasonably. Sam explained that he knew when I left that we could not go on. He wanted me to come back and sometimes he was desperate, but he knew that our relationship could never work. I recognised the pragmatic trait which had always been present in Sam's personality. Even when he seemed desperate and on the edge of madness, he had been able to centre himself, exercise surprising self-control and shift in an instant to a more balanced persona if the situation required. I had imagined him falling apart and helpless in my absence, and whilst I knew that he was genuinely upset, I now saw that the pragmatist had taken over and he had done what was necessary. Knowing that he couldn't afford to stay in our joint property he had simply found somewhere financially more viable.

Sam's flat would be available in two weeks' time. Until then, we had to find a way to live under the same roof and agree on the distribution of our possessions.

19.

Darkness before dawn

"The end goal of all this striving is to live joyfully."

Martha N. Beck

I rang Lucy, who was clearly very worried and relieved to hear from me. I had to apologise, "Lucy, I know I promised to ring and I've put you through needless anxiety, I just couldn't deal with anything except the situation at home'" I explained what had happened and the conclusion we had reached. Lucy expressed her relief and, knowing that the next couple of weeks would not be easy, made me promise that I would keep talking, let Lucy know instantly if I needed help. I knew that I would, this time there would be no broken promise.

I rang Steve. He was so pleased to hear from me. How could I explain to him that I had considered staying with Sam? My behaviour already seemed to me like complete madness. Steve had found somewhere for us to stay at the end of January, a small, cosy and secluded cottage by a river. It sounded wonderful and I couldn't wait, though it felt like a long time away and I knew there were many obstacles to overcome before then.

I also rang Julia to catch up and explain that I would not need to stay with her after all.

The next couple of weeks were harder than anything I could have imagined. Sam's rational behaviour soon disappeared. He started to hoard the things he wanted to take to his flat, forbidding me to touch them, even if I only wanted to borrow something of which I didn't have a duplicate. I found myself buying additional goods, a microwave and a vacuum cleaner, some new saucepans for Sam to take so he couldn't complain that I had something he didn't. I would do anything not to rock the boat, so desperate was I for Sam to keep his word and leave. The hostility between us was overpowering, yet I didn't dare allow it to develop into open conflict in case he threatened to stay to punish me. I was constantly on the edge, afraid to speak or act in the wrong way in case the fragile situation erupted into aggression or violence. I knew that Sam was particularly unstable during this time; the slightest provocation could send him into a rage. My fear escalated to a breathless sense of terror, my whole body was tense, I never relaxed, waking in pain and discomfort from disturbed sleep, then dragging myself to work.

I distracted myself by putting plans in place to buy Sam out of the house. Even though this would be hard, it would give me some stability whilst I decided what to do. It also meant that once I had completed the transaction, I would have no continuing legal issues to deal with and no potential disputes to face; I would be completely free.

23.

PARTING

"How peculiar endings and beginnings were. For as she latched the door behind her she found it necessary to correct herself. She was no one in particular yet. This transition was her chance to rebuild herself."

Stevie Davies, 'Four Dreamers and Emily'

It was agreed that I would stay with Lucy and Peter for a couple of days whilst Sam moved out. The day he was due to go, I packed my things and got ready to leave. Sam didn't want me to go. He became distressed and pleaded with me at least to share a sandwich with him before my journey. I agreed reluctantly and made some lunch. It was like Sam was grasping at every last second. I couldn't think what benefit there was for him in this, it seemed to upset him more. I could hardly swallow my lunch, all I wanted to do was get away, finally to experience the sense of freedom I had wanted for so long.

Half an hour later, I was at last on the road. Despite Sam's clear and genuine distress, still the only emotion I could feel was fear. It felt like I had been dominated by fear, to varying degrees, all my life. The past few weeks had simply surfaced all of that destructive emotion until I could concentrate on nothing else except the need to escape it. I craved the feeling of exhilaration I might have expected, yet it wouldn't come, only a sense of disbelief and a hypnotic shift of reality, like I was suddenly in another dimension, lost and confused.

When I reached the safety of Lucy and Peter's house, I was exhausted. I ate some dinner then went to bed, sleeping until late in the morning. The next evening, the three of us returned to my house. Sam was gone.

Within a day or so the house was transformed. We cleaned and moved furniture, lit candles and cooked delicious food. My house had rarely seen such warmth and enjoyment, it felt like a different place. To me the whole thing felt unreal, like I was dreaming and would soon wake up to find none of this was true. Despite the distorted perceptions which had led me to return home, hoping to put things right with Sam, I now knew that this was a precious chance to be free and not a single doubt about leaving Sam crossed my mind. All I could feel and think about was how close I had come to blowing my chance, condemning myself to a future of isolation and oppression. The fear still persisted and dominated, but it was becoming suffused with a sense of relief. I didn't understand what could have clouded my mind to the obvious, that my relationship had been beyond repair almost from the start and I had always had the choice to walk away.

I was beginning to recognise that the pattern of my life, of trying hopelessly to 'mend' broken and damaged relationships to my great cost, was a constant and powerful presence. It wasn't Sam I was attached to, but my pattern. Despite the strength of the support which surrounded me, the prospect of happiness for the first time in my life and the chance to break free, the pattern was like a coiled serpent within my mind. It was whispering lies and forbidding me to stray from familiar yet dangerous territory, as if that alone could offer security. It was pernicious and destructive, distracting and ever present. I knew that the danger hadn't gone with Sam's departure. The biggest challenge was within; somehow, I must learn to visualise and tame the coiled serpent, extract it from my consciousness and vaporise it before my eyes. I knew this would take time, that my battle with the serpent would continue, possibly for the rest of my life, and that its power was so strong I must seek help to tame it.

Visualising the serpent as real and independent from my consciousness for the first time, I wondered what would be left when it had been destroyed. What would this new me be like? How would I cope with life outside the serpent's comfort zone? I was so used to constraint; I had always seen my life in terms of others, working around them and trying to manage and manipulate, mould myself around their wants and needs in the false belief that this would bring happiness. What beliefs would be there to replace this pattern? I had read all the relevant books, I knew that the things I thought and felt created my reality. I began to construct elaborate representations of my consciousness. I saw the path of my life as a straight and fixed road from which I had believed I could not deviate, like a disused and overgrown railway track. I saw myself stumbling along the rails, gazing only forward, transfixed by a point in the distance which was always beyond my reach. My only goal had been to reach that point, to make my happiness materialise through exhausting and futile effort. Despite my constant struggle, the goal remained always one step ahead.

For the first time, I found myself in the present moment. The peace and freedom I had now discovered brought the opportunity of a life time. I closed my eyes and allowed the stillness to overwhelm me. I was there, simply 'in the now'. No movement was required, no dreadful longing was driving me forward. The meditation was so deep and profound my vision began to evolve spontaneously. With incredible clarity I saw myself once more on the railway track but standing still for the first time. Slowly I seemed to emerge from the trance which had caused me to walk forward at such a pace. I watched myself beginning to look around, realising that the railway track was *somewhere*. Instead of the blinkered vision which concentrated my focus on the unattainable future, I saw the overwhelming beauty of the present for the first time. I was surrounded by flowers and green fields, seagulls swooped and dived overhead, and in the distance was a grassy cliff top, beyond which I saw the sea. Despite the deep trance, I felt the warmth of tears streaming down my cheeks. How could I have missed all this beauty? I was surrounded by the endless possibilities generated by three dimensions of space and one of time. The landscape was dynamic and beautiful, powerful and compelling, a metaphor for the choice I always had but could not see. All directions were open to me, I only had to choose; I had complete freedom. All I had to do was open my mind and believe.

Later Lucy and I went to the beach. It was good to be here, actually walking on the sand rather than self-imprisoned within my car, feeling the strong wind around us, smelling the air and throwing stones into the powerful, vibrant sea. The whole world seemed to me suddenly to have come alive. In the past I seemed only to have experienced this place through the restricted vision of the goldfish bowl, as though it didn't belong to me, as though I had no right to be there. I now knew that this was only a fantasy created by the serpent in my head; the world belonged to me as much as to anyone else. We gathered shells, ran along the shore and sat on the quay, drinking coffee from paper cups. I felt a tremulous and fragile sense of relief, combined with a growing disbelief that I could so easily have denied myself all of this.

A couple of days later, Lucy and Peter went home and I was left on my own for the first time. It was strange but not frightening. I enjoyed the freedom to make my own decisions, treasured the sense of peace. I played music I hadn't heard for years, invited friends to dinner, stayed on the telephone for hours without interruption, and decorated the house. Of course, it still felt strange; often I would be out and about when a feeling of panic would overcome me, forgetting that I had no deadline, didn't need to hurry back in fear of reprisal if I was late. I still had vivid nightmares that Sam had returned, refusing to leave, and that I was once again trapped in the well.

Sam telephoned a couple of times a week. Immediately he left, he began to regret his decision. He begged my forgiveness, demanded that I give him another chance, could not understand why all his requests for contact and reconciliation were politely but firmly refused. I felt nothing except a desire to taper off my occasional contact with Sam; I now knew that nothing he said could entice me back and I knew that Sam needed to make his own decisions, carve out his own path, and that contact with me would only get in the way. I also knew that Sam was utterly sincere in his apologies and self-recrimination. With equal conviction I knew that he could never change; that no matter how many times he expressed his remorse and good intentions, the result would always have been the same. He would always be the complex, inconsistent, unpredictable Sam I had lived with for far too long.

I did not leave Sam for Steve. It is important to my story that I explain this. I believe strongly that without the love and support of my friends, family and particularly Steve, I would not have had the courage to break away. I knew intuitively that Steve and I had the chance of a life time, but the task of leaving Sam, with its complexities and inconsistencies had to be tackled itself. I do not believe that the key to breaking unhealthy patterns is to find another partner, either immediately after the end of a traumatic relationship, or whilst that relationship is still in place. As my story illustrates, that can lead to yet more poor decision making and ultimate disaster. Things simply happened the way they did for me.

A month after Sam and I separated, free from Sam at last, I spent a weekend with Steve in the cottage by the river. We were good together; we talked endlessly about the past, the fun we could have, the things we had in common. We walked in the countryside and by the river, ate in cafes and country pubs, held hands, played music and made each other laugh. Simple, everyday things, but to me they brought a sense of wonder and enchantment, as though I had never known such happiness could exist. Instinctively we knew we had all the time in the world to allow our relationship to grow. There was no rush, no desperation.

Incredibly, I had begun to realise that I could finally recognise a good guy when I met one. We agreed to meet again in a couple of weeks.

24.

RESURRECTION

*"Somewhere, something incredible
is waiting to be known."*

Carl Sagan

If this was a fairy tale, Steve and I would live happily ever after, I would instantly shake off my destructive pattern and I would have discovered the secret of a perfect life, which I would share with you.

Life, of course, is no fairy tale, though I'm privileged to say that many of my experiences do seem miraculous. As it happens, twelve years after I left Sam, Steve and I are still together and very happy, yet the simple fact of our togetherness is far from the point. The intervening years have often been tough and challenging, full of change, learning and some fatigue.

My life has changed beyond recognition. After leaving Sam I found that it was difficult to settle back into work, and within a year I applied for a new job, nearer to my family and to Steve. Although still in the same line of work, I found this job less interesting and soon applied for a further promotion. Within three years of separating from Sam, I had moved house and job twice.

Steve and I still lived a considerable distance apart and saw each other infrequently. His relationship had been faltering for some time, but its ending was tortuous. Steve admits readily that he did not handle this well, and I know that past losses had made him less clear about how to move on. Although I was secure in my knowledge that my relationship with Steve was sound, it felt like I would never have him to myself. I should have made the decision to remove myself from the situation so that it could heal, but Steve didn't want me to and I wasn't strong enough to insist. Instead, I found myself preoccupied with trying to push Steve to sort out the practical and emotional issues which remained. The situation dominated my thoughts and distracted me from other aspects of my life; I lost interest in my job and had difficulty coping with day to day responsibilities. By the time the situation finally resolved I was exhausted. Despite all I had been through, my pattern was still in charge.

My already deteriorating health began to worsen and I found the demands of my new job, which involved much travelling and long hours, too much to cope with. I began to struggle with meeting deadlines, had difficulty concentrating and found myself making mistakes. At home I found the simplest tasks too demanding. I would leave letters unopened for weeks, forgetting to deal with or respond to important business.

The years of trauma, depression, unhappiness, and now too much change and pressure, caught up with me. I struggled on for too long, until my performance at work and my health were affected. I suffered from allergies, headaches, arthritis and a range of other symptoms. Finally, I accepted a severance package and ended my lengthy career.

I badly needed relaxation and time to heal. I should have sought help with my behaviour patterns and depression and found a means of support to prevent me from falling backwards. I was financially secure and didn't need to push myself, but out of habit I found myself unable to stop; I don't think I knew how. For all my adult life I had taken too much responsibility on myself and struggled alone when there was no need.

Although it was a profound relief to be free of employment in an organisation, I still wanted to work. I started to look for work in all sorts of strange places. Deciding that my whole career must have been a mistake, I tried to become a freelance trainer and mentor in a different field-to no avail. I spent hours writing resumes, contacting anyone I thought would listen and offer me the chance to use my skills. I tried desperately to make things happen. All came to nothing. I began to believe I would never work again and became desperate to find some purpose to my life. Once again, I was looking for validation in the outside world, as though I was nothing in my own right.

Mercifully, I began to write, a childhood ambition never before realised, except in a formal and academic sense. The words came easily and brought great comfort; I came to see writing as therapeutic. When I wrote, I found the release which had evaded me. I began to realise that frantic activity pushed away the things I most desired. It had been the same all my life. When I wrote, there was peace in the moment and sometimes I found great inspiration just by banishing my thoughts. I wrote about my life and experiences, finding that a sense of understanding and clarity began to emerge almost automatically on the page. I felt I had found an inner seam of wisdom which had been dormant within me all my life, suppressed by desperation to succeed and frantic effort.

Exhausted and searching for comfort and meaning, I finally decided to look for independent outside help. I started to look for a meditation class, but nothing I came across felt right. In the end I found a holistic practitioner who possessed a range of skills. On meeting her, I felt a strong sense of connection and knew that working with her was what I needed to do. After talking to me for a while she recommended some sessions of guided meditation.

Immediately the meditation sessions brought a profound sense of relief and peace, but there was a long way to go; I had to break the habits of a life time.

I arrived at my third meditation session feeling directionless and in a bit of a state, and asked the practitioner for guidance, not really knowing what I expected. I will never forget what happened next; she looked pensive and then she said, "there's a man here, is your Dad in the spirit world?" I froze and nodded, she knew nothing of my background.

She said he had been waiting a very long time for me, he knew he hadn't listened when I was young, but he wanted me to know I was 'the apple of his eye' and he was very proud of me. Then she said, "did you write him a letter?" I burst into uncontrollable sobs. I described to her the scenario where, when I was a teenager, my father threw my letter, written to him in desperation, on the fire unopened. She said, "well, he's read it now."

She also said that he liked my partner and we were soul mates. As so many of our arguments during my teenage years were about my father's disapproval of my boyfriends, this was very important to me. She had no way of knowing any of this, but if I could have asked for anything from my father, it would have been that he was listening to me, that he was proud of me and that he approved of my partner.

What do you make of this? I can only tell you that every word is exactly as it happened. During the guided meditation that followed, I experienced a profound sense of my father's presence. The therapist guided me so far, telling me I would be taken to a place that was familiar; she then left me to experience the meditation in silence. My father and I met on the shores of a lake near to a beautiful place where we used to fly my kite when I was a child. Steve, wearing a bandanna, walked along the shore and the three of us embraced as though we were dancing together.

Afterwards I knew without doubt what this encounter meant.

The natural environment was a place where we had been the happiest, relaxed and laughing together in the years before arguments and tears.

The 'dance' reminded me of my cousin's wedding, which took place in my late adolescence. During the evening celebrations her father, (my father's brother) danced with her. Watching them together, I could clearly see how proud he was of her and how much he loved her. I felt a deep sense of sadness that my relationship with my father had deteriorated so much that we would never share such a special moment.

The shore of the lake was a reference to Carl Sagan's 'Contact', a novel about a female scientist whose beloved father dies early. She becomes the first envoy from Earth to an alien civilisation, the contact with which is made on a distant sea shore through the appearance of her dead father, who brings the great wisdom of an advanced culture. I have read this book several times, and each time I have identified with the heroin and the relationship with, and return of, her father.

Whatever the nature of my meditation experience, it felt as though my father had plundered my deepest emotions and desires, connected with my thoughts and memories, and responded with appropriateness so breath-taking its power will stay with me for the rest of my life.

After my father's early death, I believed I had lost him for good. I have difficulty describing adequately the overwhelming sense of joy I experienced at the reconciliation with him. It was much more profound than it ever could have been in life, it generated a sense of healing and self-worth I never thought I would experience, and ever since I have felt his presence as a protective force.

Two years later, the symbolism of this experience brought yet more joy and healing, but not before I was brought very close to death.

Having struggled to find my purpose after leaving work, I still also found myself ill at ease with my close relationships, at times I felt taken for granted, as though I was doing all the giving.

Steve's struggle to resolve things with his former partner had caused me immense stress and left its mark. I always knew that it was no threat to my relationship with Steve but became haunted by the lack of complete separation. Instead of allowing myself to stand back emotionally, fear and habit had kept me locked in to what was, at the time, an unhealthy situation.

I had cross words with my son over a petty and meaningless situation, but the experience damaged me deeply. He said some unkind things to me about Steve. It felt like whatever I tried to do I could never get it right. My old pattern still exerted its influence, causing me to put up with unreasonable situations for fear of being rejected.

I felt I was losing myself, my health was constantly poor and I began to suffer ear problems. I believe that all the years of struggle, of searching for meaning, depression, unhappiness, stress and too much change were catching up with me. For all I had learned, for all the undeniable progress I had made, the goal and ultimate protection of becoming my authentic self and finding a peaceful existence still eluded me.

Early in 2010, as a result of yet another ear problem, I contracted bacterial meningitis. Steve, my son, my brother and Lucy stayed with me; they were told that I would not survive. I was in intensive care for ten days and my condition was deteriorating; my friends and relatives were told to prepare for the worst. Attempts to withdraw sedation resulted in fitting and the medical staff could detect no higher brain function. It was decided that one last attempt would be made to revive me, before life support systems would be switched off and I would be allowed to "drift away". Incredibly, I came out of sedation and could respond.

No one could believe my recovery, which some see as nothing short of a miracle. I have to agree with them. This experience changed my life. It put into perspective and deeply affected my close relationships; we now value each other much more and realise what is important. My son, who had sat by my bedside with Steve for ten days, being told repeatedly that I was going to die, wrote me a wonderful letter which he thought I would never be able to read. He talked of his regret about our meaningless argument, told me how much he loved me and what I meant to him and his family, and described Steve's love and dedication to me, which he had seen when I was unconscious. He wished us a long and happy life together.

For the first time in my life, I had to stop and let go of control. I was helpless and had to recognise that my recovery would be lengthy, and the stress under which I had placed myself was completely unnecessary. It was a dangerous and dramatic way to learn that I had to rest and take care of myself. Ironically, the enforced inactivity of my period of recovery brought the greatest sense of peace I have ever known, and my life finally started to turn the corner. The pressure of trying to change the outside world to make me happy was gone, all I could do was relax and allow myself to get better. I have never felt such a sense of love and contentment. I let go of all defensiveness and realised I was safe.

As I got better, I developed some freelance work as a social work practice teacher; this work has led to other things in the field of adult education and plays to my strengths. For several years Steve and I developed and ran a successful holiday cottage business on the North Yorkshire coast. I continued to find writing a therapeutic release and means of working through challenges and preoccupations.

All of these things evolved naturally, without the frantic effort I had been used to all my working life and which I tried, unsuccessfully, to apply after leaving my former career. I love the freedom, balance and variety of these activities. Each of them draws on my knowledge and skills and brings me joy. I haven't re-invented myself by writing off my past as I initially tried to do, rather I've recognised that all my experience is valuable and makes me who I am. The strength to do these things has come from within, though it took dramatic events to bring me finally to the realisation that I had to find a peaceful space and clear my mind before my life could improve.

After my illness, Steve asked me to marry him. This was completely out of the blue, and something I never expected to happen as Steve had never been married. We had an informal wedding and each chose to wear clothes in which we felt most comfortable. Steve decided to wear a bandanna. Only later did it strike me that one of the features of the meditation in which my father appeared which had always puzzled me was the bandanna that Steve was wearing. I had never described this aspect of the meditation to Steve or to anyone else. At the time of the meditation, the prospect of us marrying had never been mentioned, yet the symbolism, combined with my poignant memories of my cousin's wedding, was so clear it reduced me to tears of joy. Not only did my father seem able to see a future for us we could never have imagined, but through the symbolism of the bandanna which Steve would wear at our future ceremony and the dance on the shores of the lake, I truly felt my father had finally danced with me at my wedding. After all those years, and despite his death, at last I knew without doubt how proud he was of me.

Whatever you believe about the nature of such experiences, for me the effect was transformational and deeply healing. It's not the medium (in the widest sense), it's the message that matters. The loss of my close relationship with my father was one of the most devastating aspects of my young life and seemed to set the disastrous pattern for my future relationships. I now believe that there were signs for many years after his death that he was trying to contact me. The message I found in his handwriting in the Bible was only one example. At a time when I was very worried about my son, a cryptic message superimposed itself on my computer screen, beginning with the words 'not in danger'; a 'lost' necklace miraculously reappeared on my bedroom carpet and many vivid dreams involving my father have turned out prophetic.

There is much more.

25.

STEVE AND ME

"...in an intimate long-term relationship, although you will experience wonderful feelings such as love and joy, you will also inevitably experience disappointment and frustration."

Russ Harris, 'The Happiness Trap'

So how is my life with Steve? A typical scenario:

"Have you moved that CD I left on the table? I wish you wouldn't move my things without asking'"

Steve is always leaving things around the place, he's so untidy; how could we have dinner on the table with his things in the way?

"I put it back in the CD rack where it belongs, I told you I was moving it but I knew you weren't listening."

"I would remember if you told me, I put it there to remind me of something I need to do later. I don't want you moving my things."

"Don't you dare tell me what to do, Steve, this is my house as well as yours and you don't respect that, it's like you just take over. I did tell you, you just don't listen. Sometimes I think I would be much better off on my own."

Why doesn't Steve listen? He's so stubborn and selfish sometimes. A few minutes later I feel a pinch on my backside.

"Ouch! Get off, I've had enough of you."

"Don't be dramatic; give us a kiss."

`No way, mate, not until you grow up."

"You know that's a vain hope. Anyway, what were we arguing about?"

I think for a second and really can't remember. I still feel angry and am now even more frustrated because I'm not sure why. Steve grabs me around the waist and begins to dance me around the kitchen, singing 'Blue Moon'.

"Fancy a glass of wine, gorgeous?"

"Quite honestly, yes."

Steve goes to get the bottle and pours us each a glass; "To you, my love and your wonderful bottom."

Still trying to resist and despite myself, I begin to giggle. I kiss Steve on the neck and we cuddle for a few minutes. It feels very safe and gentle.

Steve says, "When are you going to stop throwing yourself into a panic every time we have a cross word?" It's a good question.

It's about time I realised that even healthy relationships sometimes swoop and dive, are a patchwork of love and frustration, warmth and friction, laughter and the occasional tear. After my history of catastrophic and embittered liaisons, I was often in fear that the slightest friction was the beginning of the slippery slope.

For a long time after Sam and I parted, I went into a decline, almost to the point of depression, every time Steve and I had a cross word. I realised in my reflective moments that this was because all my relationships had started off hopeful and rewarding then degenerated into madness and hostility. I had feared that the same would happen to Steve and me; after the first year, telling myself that things were certain to deteriorate between us I had almost invited problems, over-reacting and taking the smallest hint of disruption as the beginning of the end.

I'm learning, though. And the overriding feeling I have is one of profound gratitude, even disbelief that life could be so good, turned around so dramatically. I love Steve deeply and most of the time we spend together is incredibly rewarding. I know that my feelings are reciprocated, and that I deserve his love.

Steve isn't perfect, of course, but then neither am I; who is? Our friendship developed into intimacy, with no detriment to the fun and enjoyment of our lives. In contrast to my previous pattern, where the initial excitement of romance camouflaged a lack of compatibility which later revealed itself, our common interests and enjoyment of each other's company have strengthened with time. It seems as though there is always something new to learn about each other. We explore the world together intellectually and practically, listen endlessly to music and treat each other with kindness. Occasionally we find ourselves moved to tears by the poignancy or beauty of a piece of literature, a play on the radio or a shared sentiment. It never fails to strike me as ironic that the only tears I now seem to shed are tears of joy. In my past life, I cried so much out of despair.

We also disagree vehemently sometimes, get on each other's nerves and need our own space. In other words, our relationship is quite normal. Whereas I used to believe that everyone else I knew had a perfect relationship which threw mine into stark contrast and made me feel inferior but now I recognise the tensions and frustrations which characterise all relationships. Their success or failure doesn't lie in the petty and the superficial, but in the real substance of compatibility and mutual respect.

Here is a quote from a reading I wrote for our wedding:

"I want most of all to thank my soul-mate, Steve, for his unwavering love and devotion. When I was helpless and needed you most you never left my side. You brought laughter, fun and beautiful music back into my life. You broadened my horizons and made me think about the joys and injustices of this world. Your kindness of spirit, gentle humanity and compassion for all living things inspire me and often put me to shame.

Through the peaks and troughs of life we sometimes become consumed with the petty and mundane, yet it takes so little to remind us of the strength which lies at the heart of our relationship. We have chosen to walk this path together and whatever it brings, that strength will prevail.

I love you, I admire you and I'm proud to become your wife."

26.

DEFEATING THE COILED SERPENT

"Any transition serious enough to alter your definition of self will require not just small adjustments in your way of living and thinking but a full-on metamorphosis."

Martha N. Beck

It's important for me to emphasise to you (and to myself) that life is about much more than my relationship with Steve. I preserve my independence and make sure I have my own interests. There are times when I find myself doing too much for Steve, giving too much out of fear of losing him, and taking responsibility for things alone, when they should be shared and discussed. Steve knows about the need to protect me from myself, he did his own research and sometimes raises the subject of my pattern because he knows that I could so easily slip back.

I am well aware that, despite believing that I had made progress after leaving Sam, an achievement I don't decry, my behaviour hadn't changed that much. I still failed to recognise the devastating effects of years of pain upon my mind and body and took no protective action against the dysfunction that remained within my life. I now realise that I was suffering from post traumatic stress disorder which affected and effectively ended my long-term career. Had I sought help at the time and had there been some understanding of this from within my organisation, things might have been different. In the end, though, all that happened was ultimately for the best.

The impact of serious illness on my relationships changed my life forever, though I know that the most fundamental change is within me and about the respect I have for myself; that is the greatest protection I can have.

I still remember with horror my inability to break away from Sam, and the way I almost turned my back on the opportunity to transform my life. I can't be complacent, I know that my pattern is ingrained, that I should always remain on my guard for signs that I might be losing my sense of balance and proportion. The dramatic effects of negative experience such as my illness eventually fade and the ordinary takes over. In that context it is easy to forget how far I have come and the lessons I have learned.

If you have experienced abuse you will probably have encountered others who can't understand why some of us repeat past mistakes, who believe that we want to be mistreated and fail to see that all our energy is spent trying to stop the abuse rather than enjoying it in some perverse way. It's just that people who are vulnerable often try to *mend* broken relationships, constantly attempting to recapture the initial sense of excitement rather than realising that the effort is futile, that they need to walk away.

If you were to ask how I can claim to have overcome my self-destructive life pattern, when I found it so hard to leave my abusive partner and even when that relationship ended I still found myself preoccupied with trying to change unhealthy situations and enduring unnecessary pain, you would be asking a pertinent question. My response is that I was still entrenched in my pattern and that change, as I have observed, is a slow process; there is no panacea. My salvation came during the rare and precious times when I was able to surrender, clear my mind and allow my life to evolve, in contrast to the many times when I tried to make things happen.

For me, this was a spiritual as well as a practical process. For example, the time I sat in my car after the "in silence we can know

God" message, the enforced peacefulness following serious illness when I could do nothing else but surrender and the meditation about the railway track during which I stopped and saw, for the first time, the world around me and its potential. These instances were followed by profound change and healing which had nothing to do with my pattern of frantic searching for a solution. It may be counter-intuitive to see doing nothing and surrendering control as the key to progress, however I have come to realise that it is the *essential* component in healing destructive life patterns, escaping traumatic bonding and valuing one's self.

Even without a spiritual component, in a purely pragmatic sense the simple act of stopping and clearing our minds allows us to see the wider picture and recognise that we are in control and can make choices about our lives. This is a right of all human beings but one which sometimes becomes obscured by our complex interactions, especially if we are vulnerable.

What advice would I give to you if you are struggling with relationships? I know it is hard to gain insight and break away, that the slightest hint of affirmation, perceived or real, can throw you into a vortex of over-reaction, believing that your partner has finally changed for the better. In order to get help, you should find someone who can identify or work with your behaviour patterns, you should read the right books, find some peace from meditation or solitude; preferably a mixture of these and whatever works for you. I would tell you that no matter how constrained you feel, how attached to your home or their possessions, no matter how hopeless your situation seems, nothing is worth the terrible imprisonment which results from abusive relationships and their toxic effects. I have learned from many years of suffering, and a close brush with death, that living with an unhealthy pattern can bring about serious mental and physical illness.

I would tell you that there is always help at hand. I know it is hard to reveal the distressing secrets of abusive relationships to others, I understand well the shame and dishonour, the sense of unbearable exposure. I have felt it myself, yet when I think back, everyone I told had understood, been eager to support me in breaking free. I now know that there is always help to be had, you only have to ask.

It's for these reasons that I've developed a programme to help you to overcome the kinds of challenges I've faced. The exercises at the end of this book are simply a taster, if you would like to know more and you are interested in taking part in either a group or a retreat, please feel free to contact me-my details are at the end of this book.

Can I promise a happy ending and everlasting love? The answer is complex. In the end I'm lucky, even if my luck is hard won, gained despite myself. But it took me so long, years of struggle and suffering that I could have escaped at any moment if I had just had the insight to see that I deserved better. The struggle very nearly killed me.

I can't promise a perfect partner, a harmonious relationship waiting in the wings, nor do I see this as the real point. I know from my own experience that even when the opportunity to engage in a healthy and balanced partnership presents itself, it can so easily be destroyed by the whispering of the coiled serpent. The real triumph for me is the change within myself, the increased calmness and greater self-respect, the absence of defensiveness and a healthier perspective on life and relationships. I know that this change is necessary for all who crave love and affirmation from the outside world but love themselves too little.

There is no magic potion which brings about instant transformation, which delivers the happy ever after. Without the gradual reconstruction of self-respect and liking, even self-love, danger will still lurk. I have always shied away from the concept of "loving oneself", seen it as an egotistical and arrogant concept, sentimental and idealised. I now know that it is an essential ingredient in the taming of the serpent, that only when I believed that I was worthy of genuine and unconditional love, did I attract it from the outside world. I can assure you, my fellow travellers, of one thing, if you are able to recognise your self-worth you will at last be discerning about relationships, able to resist the sense of panic at the thought of being alone, less desperate for affirmation from outside, because it is present within. And you will know when something is working and when it isn't; you will know a good person when you meet one-and so much more about what is good and not so good in

119

your lives.

Mine is certainly a love story with a happy ending, but in much more than the conventional sense. I have learned to ask myself whether I would allow a precious child to be treated in the way I have treated myself. I know that the challenge is always to think of myself as that precious child, and remember that I am as worthy of respect, love and protection as anyone else.

We make one journey through this fragile and precious life. No one can intrude upon that journey without our permission. If the wrong people ride along with us, mocking and laughing, making us unhappy and causing us pain, it is because we allow them on board. At any point we can change direction, breathe the air and savour the peace. What is the virtue in constantly driving ourselves forward, always trying to make things happen, if the result is so much suffering?

Time and time again, through relationships with men, I believed I had re-discovered the feeling of love and safety provided by the relationship with my father in my early childhood. When it all fell apart, I tried tirelessly to reason and restore, as though I was still a powerless child, pleading futilely with my father to listen, to become again the wise and gentle dad he once had been. The urge to repeat this pattern was so strong, it blinded me to the fact that I was free, an independent adult who had the choice to walk away.

It was difficult to see how, as a child, I could have changed these events which so dominated and shaped my life. Yes, I was a difficult teenager, isn't that natural? Don't all children reach the stage where they fight for independence? The power differential between adult and child places a responsibility upon parents to handle such challenges with love, or they can so easily end in disaster. As a teenager I experienced my father's behaviour as harsh and punitive, designed to crush my spirit; only as an adult reviewing these events can I now see his actions as a misguided attempt to protect me.

Above all, I wanted my father to be proud of me, and in the most miraculous way he has confirmed that he is. Even beyond death, I believe he tries to protect me, but now in a very different way. I want him to be reassured that no one will ever hurt me so deeply again, that, with his help, I have learned to bring into being the thing he so desired but could not achieve in life; the protection of his precious child.

To my readers, no doubt fellow travellers on this painful and dangerous road, I wish you love and fulfilment, I wish you peace, and above all I wish you respect for and belief in yourself.

27.

REFLECTIONS

"I mistrust anyone who offers constant happiness, endless success, instant confidence, or effortless self-growth."

David K Reynolds, 'Playing Ball on Running Water'

This is the story of my life so far, but I have no doubt that its challenges are far from over, that the sleeping coiled serpent in my head is waiting for an opportunity to whisper its venomous instructions. I know I will always need to be on my guard, know where to find help, and in touch with my spiritual side for guidance.

Do I see myself as a victim? Not at all. Apart from the experiences of my childhood, I had the choice to change things at any moment. The overpowering influence of my life pattern prevented me from recognising or exercising that choice. I do, however, forgive myself for my omission. Even for people whose lives have been far more balanced and secure it can be difficult to make drastic life changes. Now I constantly remind myself of what I have overcome and what I have achieved. I can spot the influence of my pattern and deal with its excesses before they take hold. I now know that being my authentic self is the most powerful thing I can be, far more attractive than the woman who dedicated her life to changing or pleasing others out of the desperate pursuit of happiness.

For much of my life I didn't really know or respect myself. Buried beneath the weight of defensiveness and the need for approval from the outside world was a strong and capable woman who knew exactly what she wanted, and what she had to give. Yet I made the most disastrous decisions because, at crucial times in my life, I listened to others, forgot, or didn't know how, to consult my true self and ask for spiritual guidance, and became seduced by false promises.

In order to be truly happy, a state which I believe has nothing to do with idealised notions of true love and a perfect life, one has to possess intimate self-knowledge. Without this knowledge, the resulting uncertainty generates poor life decisions, overwhelming stress and constant struggle. I will not pretend this knowledge is easy to come by, especially for people whose early life experience robs them of the confidence and self-belief which would otherwise help them to know and respect themselves. My story is a poignant illustration of that struggle.

I am sceptical of the counsel of perfection offered by many self-help authors, whose promises of radical life change rest on mantras, "cosmic ordering", positive thinking and the like. Without fundamental re-building of confidence, life improvements simply will not come, and vulnerable people may follow such advice, make daring decisions and radical changes, only to find themselves devastated by yet more failure and rejection.

For many, many years I read every self-help book on the shelf, confusing myself with conflicting advice and techniques, and misinterpreting "signs" and events, leading me down false trails and into poor decisions. Many people with similar life experiences to mine take the same path. I have expressed my reservations about these things, yet there is an undeniable element to my life which is spiritual; both intellectually and intuitively I have a spiritual connection. In western culture, conventional religion is often (but not always) detached from this aspect of connection with the numinous, and we have become dependent as a society on physical manifestation in a concrete world. Those who will doubt this aspect of my story or who seek absolute scientific proof may or may not find it, I would simply ask them to respect the valid and powerful testimony of others whose genuine and often unsolicited experiences leave them in no doubt that there is a spiritual dimension which sustains us after death and can enrich our lives on Earth.

I have learned to understand, to welcome and to work with my innate spirituality. I am still drawn to esoteric works but find myself more discerning. I have also learned to develop and trust my own perspective, which is simple and clear. As I have come to understand more clearly my preferences, skills and beliefs, I have also learned to make deeper spiritual connections. It is still sometimes hard not to misinterpret, and I find myself often confusing thought and intuition, though I now see this as part of the journey, and the more I work with my experiences, the more adept I become at integrating my intellectual and spiritual proclivities.

So, who am I? The best way to describe my journey towards self-knowledge is to look at my mistakes, and they encompass far more than my personal relationships. For instance, for many years I worked in an organisation. Although there were times when I loved and worked well at my job, there were just as many times when I felt demoralised, confined and unhappy. Every role I had, I tried to adapt to suit my personality without stopping to analyse that this meant I might be doing the wrong job. Looking back, right from early adolescence I was drawn to creative thought and self-expression. The philosophy and counter-culture of the sixties appealed to me deeply and I loved literature and drama, comparative religion and popular science. At school I received poor advice on subject choice and career direction, choosing subjects because my friends took them, or because my father would have chosen them. I had a natural tendency towards science, particularly physics, but was dissuaded from that course because I was not strong enough at maths. Looking back, this saddens me greatly because I believe that with a little extra tuition I could have followed my interest. I was persuaded to take biology as I was seen as a "people person" and failed miserably as it simply didn't interest me. It seemed not to have occurred to the careers teacher that people skills, writing skills and physics might be compatible. When I now read my favourite popular science authors such as Lee Smolin and Joao Magueijo, free thinkers who combine an anarchic approach with a philosophical and analytical perspective, producing wonderful and inspiring commentaries on modern physics, I despair at the advice I received.

At university I found myself enjoying astronomy and philosophy over and above my social work studies, yet I followed the latter route as it was vocational and would help me to find employment. My natural tendency was towards free expression and I loved teaching and training, finding creative ways to help adults learn. Given this description of my natural preferences and tendencies, it was ironic that I should find myself employed by a bureaucratic organisation which inevitably demanded conformity and obedience, two traits which had never been my strong points! Yet my career decisions were based on much more than poor advice. Again, my desire to please others by achieving conventional success, combined with my lack of self-knowledge, led me to engage in a lengthy career which was far from ideal for a free-spirited creative thinker. Instead I constantly tried to adapt the job to suit me. As a result, I sometimes found myself struggling with the demands of my employers, at times subjected to extreme bullying, and my health and wellbeing suffered greatly. I should have realised that what was painful wasn't working and walked away. Destructive life patterns apply to all areas of life.

That this same passionate free thinker should also find herself trapped for lengthy periods in destructive and repressive relationships is tragic. My first marriage, although ill-matched, stormy and unhappy, was less confining and my husband always supported me in my achievements. My second marriage, however, robbed me of all joy and self-respect.

I stayed for more than ten years with a man who demanded conformity to ideals I despised, disapproved of and successfully repressed my tendency towards self-expression and rubbished my achievements. As I write this, I am still thinking "How could I?" I can only answer that, from the privileged perspective of my current life, it seems so clear that this relationship was wrong in every way. The signs were there right from the beginning. I am also now able to understand comprehensively why an intelligent woman with every opportunity to take stock of her life, and time to understand herself, should become so consumed with a dysfunctional relationship in the pursuit of security, outside approval and respectability. I was repeating the patterns of my childhood, trying desperately to get back to the safety and protection of my loving Dad, who deserted me in my teens.

It may be surprising to hear that I don't regret my life. Every painful experience has brought powerful learning. My struggle to prove myself has equipped me with a wide range of knowledge and experience and the pain I have felt has propelled me on a journey to understand myself, and to acquire a little wisdom I am able to share, in the hope that others may benefit. Had my life been happy and secure, resulting in wise choices and a comfortable existence, I would have had little motivation to explore the complexities of human interaction which have inspired me so much.

From the vantage point of my happy, but still challenging, life I feel privileged and grateful for the richness of my experience.

THE HALL
OF
MIRRORS:

Exercises for Adopting
Healthier Life Patterns

EXERCISE 1:

THE ORIGIN OF LIFE PATTERNS

Take some 'time out' to think about your life patterns and how they originated.

Did you experience trauma, loss, sadness or disappointment which caused you to look for happiness elsewhere, only to find that your new relationship was just as unhappy?

What were you trying to put right?

Write or draw your life pattern and keep it to refer to as you work through later exercises.

EXERCISE 2:

YOUR LIFE NOW

Draw a picture or a write a few paragraphs about your life as it is now. Include your relationships, work, hobbies, activities, pets, where you live, in fact anything that seems relevant.

- If some of your relationships are unhappy, think about how your life pattern may have played a part, or prevented you from caring for and protecting yourself.

- Think back to the previous exercise and remind yourself of the way your life pattern emerged.

- Were you seeking to put something right or to re-create a relationship from your early life?

- Keep the exercise to refer to as you build a picture of your life.

Exercise 3:

STOP

Use the following STOP exercise to allow your subconscious mind to process what you have written or drawn.

Find a space which is comfortable, sit quietly and calmly for a few minutes and clear your mind. Don't try to suppress or manage your thoughts, just allow them to be, and try to observe them from afar. Breathe normally and listen to each breath; let your subconscious mind find some breathing space. Sit like this for a while, then open your eyes slowly and take a breath in and out.

When you have finished walk around for a while, go outside if possible and notice everything about your environment; the temperature, other people, growing things, streets, pavements and sounds. Try to avoid using technology for a while after this experience so you can stay connected to the four-dimensional world.

Use this exercise often as you work through your story.

Exercise 4:

Positive Relationships

Think of a relationship you experienced which was or is positive. This could be any relationship, a life partner, a child, a family member, a teacher, a friend a neighbour etc.

- Write about or draw what was or is good about this relationship

- Think about how you met or how your relationship began

- Think about what made or makes you compatible with this person. What was it in you that made a connection with them?

- Write about or draw how the relationship made or makes you feel

- What values and beliefs did or do you share with this person?

- How did or does this person treat you?

Use the STOP exercise to allow your subconscious to process what you have written or drawn.

Exercise 5:

Who are
You?

This time either write or draw yourself without reference to relationships with other people:

- Think about the things that matter to you, things you care about and your likes and dislikes.

- Try to recall times when you have been moved to tears by an experience, inspired by something or encouraged to take action in support of a cause.

- Think about what makes you laugh and things you used to do which you miss.

- When you have done this, write a paragraph or draw a picture of the person you have re-discovered. You now have an emerging picture of your authentic self.

Use the STOP exercise to allow your subconscious to process what you have written or drawn.

Exercise 6:

What do You want to Happen?

This time, building on the previous exercises where you have identified your life pattern, reviewed your relationships and started to uncover your authentic self, think of something you want to change about your life and relationships and which you find difficult to tackle;

- Remind yourself of the reasons you want things to change, for example, is someone cruel or uncaring? Are you being physically harmed? Are you being isolated from the people you love or the things you want to do?

- Allow yourself to experience the emotional impact of this situation. If you are being harmed emotionally or physically, write about or draw the impact on yourself and others and notice the feelings this evokes. Sit quietly with your eyes closed and allow your subconscious to process what is happening.

- Imagine yourself free from this situation-how will you feel? What will you be able to do that you can't do now? How may making this change benefit others in your life?

- Decide on one step you can take to change things; this could be as simple as telling someone how you feel, asking for help and support or as significant as deciding to leave the situation altogether.

- Remember that you and those you love have the right to a safe and peaceful life and that at any moment you can decide to take action towards that goal

Use the STOP exercise to allow your subconscious to process what you have written or drawn.

EXERCISE 7:

WHAT DO YOU DESERVE?

Take some time to think about the previous exercises; you could make a list of all the things you have discovered about yourself and review it, draw a picture or clear your mind and let the image of your authentic self-emerge

Describe the relationships you feel you deserve-include all kinds of relationships, for example, with wider family members, an employer or with a life partner

- What would these relationships feel like?

- What would you have in common with the people in these relationships?

- What values and beliefs would you share?

- What would you be able to do?

Use the STOP exercise to allow your subconscious to process what you have written or drawn.

EXERCISE 8:

SELF-COMPASSION

Behaving compassionately towards yourself is a vital ingredient in recovering from abusive or unhappy situations. Recognising that you are worthy of love and protection depends on this process-especially if your life pattern began with past trauma:

- Write about or draw a representation of your strengths, beliefs and interests, include the things you have achieved which give you joy.

- Next write about or draw a representation of the challenges you have faced and the steps you have taken to overcome them. Remember that all your experiences have helped you to learn and grow as a human being.

- Sit quietly and let your thoughts come and go, concentrating on your breathing.

- Imagine yourself surrounded by love and protection. Recognise that you are as entitled to these things as anyone else and congratulate yourself on the journey you have taken.

When future challenges come, remember what you have achieved and remind yourself that it is more powerful to let go of the struggle and to look inside for the strength and compassion you now know to be there

Use the STOP exercise to allow your subconscious to process what you have written or drawn.

EXERCISE 9:

WRITE YOUR STORY

Finally, write, draw or represent your story in whatever form feels right:

- Start with whatever events seem most influential.

- Describe the challenges and situations you faced and your reactions to them; think about why you reacted as you did and express the emotions you felt.

- If it was difficult to make decisions or to break away from unhappy situations, reflect on why this was and what you couldn't see or do at the time.

- Describe how and why things changed for you, or if you are still trapped by your life pattern, describe how you could break free given what you have learned about yourself and who could help.

Sit quietly and concentrate on your breathing; let your thoughts come and go and ask for guidance. Know that you are free and can choose to change your life at any time.

About the Author

Kath Twigg is social work trained. She spent a long career in the criminal justice system where she worked as a practitioner, manager and senior manager. Currently she works as a freelance university lecturer, mentor, trainer and writer. She also runs therapeutic writing courses for survivors of domestic abuse and workshops for those who wish to escape destructive life patterns and abusive relationships. She lives very happily with her husband in the Peak District of Derbyshire.

Kath Twigg has devised a powerful group programme to help you to adopt healthier life patterns. She can offer retreats and courses tailored to your needs. Kath can be contacted on:

Kathtwigg2@gmail.com
www.kathtwigg.com

Suggested Further Reading:
Thich Nhat Hanh: "Silence"
Russ Harris: "The Happiness trap"
Martha Beck: "Diana Herself"
Stevie Davies: "Four Dreamers and Emily"
Gillie Bolton: "Write Yourself"
Oliver Burkeman: "The Antidote: Happiness for People who can't Stand Positive Thinking"
Robin Norwood: Women Who Love Too Much

Lightning Source UK Ltd.
Milton Keynes UK
UKHW02f0646180818
327416UK00006B/489/P